Simply
SUGAR FREE

SUE BROWN

Simply Sugar Free

6 Simple Steps to Conquer Sugar Addiction

By Sue Brown

The content of this book is for general instruction only. Each person's physical and emotional condition is unique. The instruction in this book is not intended to replace or interrupt the reader's relationship with a physician or other professional. Please consult your doctor for matters pertaining to your specific health and diet.

Published By:

www.PromotingNaturalHealth.com

Printed in the United States of America

ISBN-10: 0990646246
ISBN-13:978-0-9906462-4-2

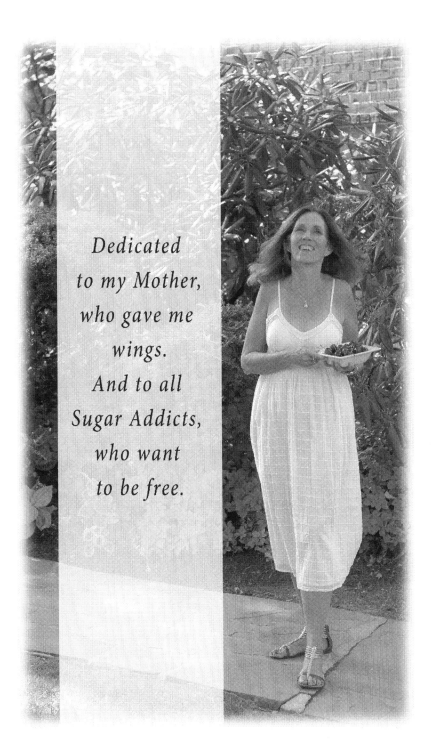

Dedicated
to my Mother,
who gave me
wings.
And to all
Sugar Addicts,
who want
to be free.

Table of Contents

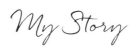

Hello, my name is Sue. And I'm a recovered Sugar Addict.

I lost 52 pounds in 52 weeks when I was 52. But mine is not a story of weight loss. It is a story of recovery. From a lifelong struggle with Sugar Addiction. I now live at the intersection of neuroscience and nutrition.

It can be a messy, confusing place. Some days the Vegans and Paleos collide head-on. Or low-carb fanatics flame low-fat fanatics in cyberspace. Take a trip to a bookstore and you'll see what I mean. We don't suffer from too little information. We suffer from too much.

But once you understand that we're all different and that ultimately no one knows what's best for you except for YOU, you can pick yourself up from the wreckage and begin to figure it out. One step at a time.

No drugs. No surgery. No kidding.

Many people have gone down this path before me. To them I am grateful for shining a light into what was complete darkness for me for most of my life.

Many more people are travelling the path with me now right now. And to them I am grateful as well. Science is advancing at such a rapid pace that it is increasingly enlightening and confusing, all at the same time.

The more information there is, the more loose ends there are to tie up.

Much of the research is occurring in very narrow silos. Neuroscience. Biochemistry. Pediatric Endocrinology. Physiology. Cognitive Behavioral Therapy. Neuropharmacology. Even Orthopedics.

Unfortunately, we don't exist in narrow silos. We exist in busy, chaotic and often stressful lives. We don't have time to connect the dots between the disciplines…even if those connections could unlock the mystery of ourselves. (It did for me.)

I've always known that my weight problem was in my head, not my body. That sugar delivered great "highs" and moments of intense clarity and inspiration – and comfort.

As a child at breakfast I heaped sugar on Frosted Flakes and washed it all down with Tang. After all, if it was good enough for astronauts it must be good enough for me. At lunch I shunned cold cuts for PB&J on Wonder bread. Dinner was usually mac & cheese or spaghetti.

That's a 100% carb day, recipe for an epic fail.

But that's what I wanted. What I craved. My hard-working but poor single mother was doing the best she could, unwittingly caught in the trap between a sugar-craving child and a food industry that was (and still is…) happy to accommodate those cravings in the name of profit.

Along the way I went from comforting myself with sugar to using it like a drug, unable to stop. It helped me cope with what I would come to know and love as my highly-sensitive personality, a tendency toward introversion and a relentless creative drive.

It was during a "Sugar Blues" workshop when my weight was at its highest (191 pounds on my 5'4" frame to be exact) that I began to unravel the mystery of sugar's effects on me. When my company offered a financial incentive for healthy activities a few months later, my first phone call was to the Health Coach who delivered the workshop. For the next six months we worked one-on-one. We tackled food issues but, more importantly, we explored ways to nourish myself in non-food ways such as meditation and creative visualization.

Fast forward seven years.

Now I am a Health Coach, too, having graduated from the Institute for Integrative Nutrition. I work with individual clients and groups to unravel THEIR issues with sugar. It's my way of giving back…to be more than a dream of nectar, but the fruit on the tree. Using my experience to make a difference in other peoples' lives.

> *"Before I die, grant me one thing.*
>
> *Grant one thing to me.*
>
> *Don't let me dream of nectar.*
>
> *Make me fruit on the tree."*

Abigail Washburn, Lyrics
"Dreams of Nectar" from the album City of Refuge

P.S. I haven't gained back a pound in seven years. Because once your blood sugar and brain chemistry are balanced, you don't need sweets to nourish you – physically or emotionally. Just real, whole food. The way Mother Nature intended.

I'm a journalist by training. I enjoy digesting complex topics and simplifying them. In this book I have deliberately over-simplified many things, as a favor to you. You don't need the gory details, just enough information to start making better decisions, on your own. Or with the guidance of a Health Coach.

I've also gone on to study the psychology and sociology of how people and organizations change (or not!). Turning these skills inward resulted in the process I used for my personal transformation. And that I'm sharing with you now.

My goal is to give you a map to help you navigate my neighborhood, that intersection of neuroscience and nutrition. I don't have THE answer for anyone. No one does.

But what I do have is a proven process to guide you through the intersections…the decisions you have to make every minute of every hour of every day …of what to eat and how to nourish yourself.

Yours to a fruitful life,

Sue

P.P.S.

Although this book is focused on Sugar Addiction and not weight loss, most Sugar Addicts find that weight loss is one of the biggest benefits of overcoming Sugar Addiction.

To that end, I've included research throughout this book that comes from the National Weight Control Registry (NWCR), of which I am a proud member.

Given that few individuals succeed at long-term weight loss, the NWCR was established in 1994 by Rena Wing, Ph.D. from Brown Medical School, and James O. Hill, Ph.D. from the University of Colorado, to identify and investigate the characteristics of individuals who have succeeded at long-term weight loss.

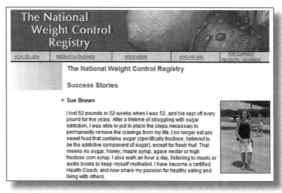

More than 6,000 people (including me) are members of the registry. All of the members have maintained a weight loss of at least 30 pounds for more than one year.

Detailed questionnaires and annual follow-up surveys are used to examine the behavioral and psychological characteristics of weight maintainers, as well as the strategies they use to maintain their weight losses.

For additional research results or to join the registry, visit the NWCR website at http://www.nwcr.ws/.

Sugar and Addiction
The Nitty Gritty Details

This Chemistry Matters

Don't let your eyes glaze over!

I know, I know. The last thing you want is a chemistry lesson. You want a quick fix. You want to lose weight NOW.

But trust me on this.

This chemistry matters. It could change your life!

I know. Because my life changed forever the moment I understood that I was addicted to sugar. Fructose, in particular.

I had tried every diet under the sun. Counting calories. Counting points. Eating nothing but fruit until noon. Not eating fruit, ever. Low fat, high carb. Then the opposite.

Sometimes I would be determined, follow the rules and lose weight. But I always gained back what I lost. And more. Like everyone else who tries. I couldn't sustain the restrictions I forced upon myself. My cravings trumped my willpower.

I couldn't make it from breakfast to lunch without making "bad" choices. Crap. Why was that so? I was motivated. I "knew" what to do.

Then I learned that sugar is addictive. And once I could trace my cravings all the way to the source, I found food freedom.

Because when you know what you CAN'T eat, you also know what you CAN eat!

I am a Fructose Fanatic, driven by the nearly instant "high" that sweet foods deliver directly from my taste buds to my brain. A signal as strong as cocaine. Now, you might be a Glucose Glutton, driven to eat starches for the blood sugar rush that trips YOUR pleasure switch.

Either way, a better understanding of what's going on in your brain and your body when you're craving "sugar" or "carbs" will help you fuel your body without tripping your addiction switch.

What's the difference between having a sweet tooth and being a sugar addict?

A person with a sweet tooth can eat one chocolate chip cookie, enjoy it and stop. A sugar addict can't.

A lot of people I talk with describe themselves as "emotional eaters". I get that. I thought I was one, too. But when you better understand the underlying biochemistry of addiction you might see that it's not emotion driving you ... it's a force much larger than that.

Nine out of 10 people see food as food. That's it. Nothing more. They might "occasionally" over eat or binge. But it's no big deal. And the urge passes.

But one in 10 of us gets hooked. Maybe even from the first bite. When an urge to eat comes over us, it doesn't go away. It gets a hold of our primal instinct to survive and demands that we eat. And eat. And eat again.

> *"No one can exert a cognitive inhibition, willpower, over a biochemical drive that goes on every minute, of every day, of every year."*
>
> Dr. Robert Lustig, author of
> *"Fat Chance: Beating the Odds Against Sugar, Processed Food, Obesity, and Disease"*

While we're talking numbers did you know that currently just a third of people are normal weight? Another third is overweight and the remaining third is obese? What? Two-thirds of us are overweight or obese?!?! When did we get so fat?!

P.S. It's likely that many of the overweight and obese people are sugar addicts and don't even know it! The same holds true for the growing number of people with Type 2 Diabetes. They may be sugar addicted and not even know!

Where did it all begin?

As children we were soothed, bribed and rewarded with food.

Over the years, an intricate network of brain systems and neurotransmitters encoded these experiences deep in our brains -- connecting our reward center, the part of the brain that makes us feel pleasure, to our memory centers that remember how great the reward felt.

Each time we were stressed and ate comforting foods, those connections became stronger. Eventually they became unconscious responses that prime us for addictive behaviors. Things that we feel compelled to repeat over and over again.

Your conscious mind knows what you need to do—avoid sugar and exercise, for example—but sometimes your unconscious mind has the upper hand.

For me, my unconscious mind always won when it had addiction on its side.

But no more.

Stick with me. One step at a time, we can conquer this.

Sugar 101

There are as many as 56 names for sugar. So if you're confused about "sugar" no wonder.

So let's start simply -- just talking about what we think of as "sugar" – the white stuff we sprinkle on top of or into other foods.

Table sugar is technically called sucrose and is a disaccharide (two simple sugars, a.k.a. monosaccharides). It looks like this:

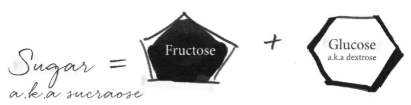

See, it's confusing already! We've got three aliases and we're just getting started.

I promise you, it gets even more confusing. But I'll do my best to simplify things in the interest of helping you unravel your sugar issues for yourself.

To truly understand sugar addiction, next we need to dissect this disaccharide into its individual components: fructose and glucose. Because they act dramatically differently in our bodies and our brains. Both can be addictive, but in different ways.

Glucose 101

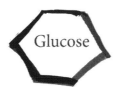

Glucose is the "good" sugar molecule, relatively speaking.

It is the main power supply for most cells, and is the only energy supply that certain cells can use (like brain and red blood cells).

Glucose is carried to the cells through the bloodstream via the transporting hormone insulin.

Glucose in our blood (a.k.a. blood sugar) is fuel, like gasoline is to a car. It supplies energy to all the cells in our bodies via our blood. Normal blood sugar is slightly less than one teaspoon of sugar in your body's five or so quarts of blood.

Here's how it works:

As we digest sugars and starches, our blood sugar rises.

When it does, our pancreas releases insulin to transport the blood sugar to our cells, hoping to find cells that need some glucose.

- Our brain, for one, needs a regular supply.
- If we've been active, more of the sugar is likely to be wanted by cells, including our many muscle cells.

As more and more glucose is absorbed into our cells, our blood sugar levels come down. Any extra glucose is stored as glycogen (a.k.a. stored glucose) in the liver and muscles.

Blood sugar tends to settle down about an hour after a meal (depending on the size of the meal and the kinds of food eaten).

- Sugars and starches raise insulin faster and higher than proteins or fats.
- The greater the fiber content of a meal, the slower insulin rises and the more controlled the process is.

Here is what this looks like. The solid line is blood sugar. The dotted line is the insulin response.

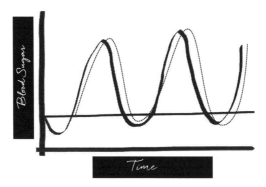

If you eat the right amount of food for your physical activity level, then blood sugar always has some place healthy to go; insulin rises and falls in a controlled manner.

But when insulin has more blood sugar than your cells need, the insulin stimulates production of triglycerides, which can become stored fat. This is how you gain weight.

If you continually eat too much and gain weight, your cells get tired of seeing insulin come driving up to their door to drop off more glucose than they need. In fact, they shutter their windows and lock their doors. Your cells become insulin resistant.

With nowhere for the glucose to go, your blood sugar continues to rise, insulin resistance gets worse, cholesterol levels go up, blood pressure goes up, triglyceride levels go up, and inflammation starts heating up. Eventually this leads to Type 2 Diabetes, along with many risk factors for heart disease.

Fructose 101

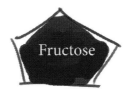

OK, so glucose is essentially good and essential to life.

Fructose, on the other hand, is not. You might call it the evil twin. Or the "f" word.

Historically we only consumed fructose when fruit was in season. That's because fructose, a.k.a. fruit sugar, is found primarily in fresh fruit.

> **Whereas every cell in our body can use glucose, our liver is the only organ that can metabolize fructose in significant amounts.**
>
> **Fructose can't be used by our cells for energy.**

If we got fructose only from fresh fruit, we'd be OK. But today most of the fructose in the Standard American Diet (a.k.a. S.A.D., so sad!) comes not from fresh fruit, but from sugar and High Fructose Corn Syrup (a.k.a. HFCS) in soft drinks and highly processed foods.

Fructose is intensely sweet, more than twice as sweet as glucose.

When fructose touches the taste receptors on your tongue, opioids are released in your brain. These opioids, which are like natural pain killers or endorphins, trigger the release of dopamine, the chemical that's responsible for feelings of pleasure. Your brain remembers the pleasure you get from sugar so that you will come back for more.

We are all wired to find sweets attractive. After all, in the caveman days eating sweets helped us build up stores of fat to survive the winter. But some of us, which we'll talk about later, are overly-sensitive to the taste of sweet. So we don't eat just enough to survive. We eat what we need to survive, but addiction takes hold and we can't stop.

As you digest food containing fructose, the fructose lands in your liver and kicks off a series of complex chemical transformations.

- The liver uses fructose, a carbohydrate, to create fat in a process called lipogenesis.
- Tiny fat droplets begin to accumulate in your liver cells and create non-alcoholic fatty liver disease (a.k.a. NAFLD), which looks just like the livers of people who drink too much alcohol. Get it? Fructose has the same effect on the liver as alcohol…without the buzz!
- Some of the fat ends up in your blood as small dense LDL that lodges in blood vessels, causing atherosclerosis and, subsequently, heart attacks.

The good news is that the fructose that naturally occurs in fruit is generally considered to be OK. Fruit is self-limiting in that you'll get full from the fiber and water in the fruit before you can eat enough to be dangerous to your health.

According to the Harvard Heart Letter, the breakdown of fructose in the liver does more than lead to the build up of fat.[1]

It also:

- Elevates triglycerides
- Increases harmful LDL (so-called bad cholesterol)
- Promotes the buildup of fat around organs (visceral fat)
- Increases blood pressure
- Makes tissues insulin resistant, a precursor to diabetes
- Increases the production of free radicals, energetic compounds that can damage DNA and cells.

And because fructose is the sweetest naturally-occurring carbohydrate… enter its addictive properties.

When rats were allowed to choose between water sweetened with sucrose (half glucose/half fructose) or cocaine the majority of animals preferred the sweet taste of sucrose.

The researcher's conclusion: The intense sweetness can surpass cocaine reward, even in drug addicts![2]

A side note for diabetics here. Sweeteners high in fructose (such as agave nectar) are often recommended for diabetics because they don't spike blood sugar. True that. But if you're wired as a Fructose Fanatic you can still become addicted to the fructose and find weight loss a frustrating venture.

Starch 101

Often when I talk about my addiction to sugar, clients and friends give me a blank stare.

"Sue, it's not sweets that I crave. It's pasta, bagels and potatoes."

Aha! These "starchy" foods are just a bunch of glucose molecules strung together. When they're broken apart in the digestion process, they're just sugar. And can trigger Sugar Addiction.

If you crave starches, you're what I call a Glucose Glutton. Here's what that looks like:

Starch =
Up to 100 or
more glucose
molecules
⟨ Glucose ⟩ + ⟨ Glucose ⟩ + ⟨ Glucose ⟩

Let's take a look at what happens when fructose and glucose are digested.

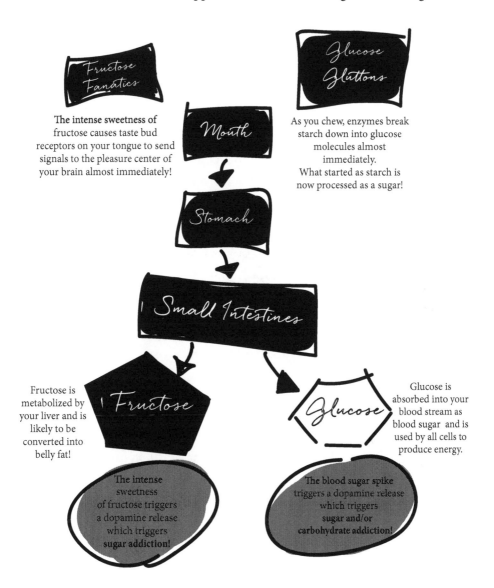

Fructose Fanatics

The intense sweetness of fructose causes taste bud receptors on your tongue to send signals to the pleasure center of your brain almost immediately!

Glucose Gluttons

As you chew, enzymes break starch down into glucose molecules almost immediately.
What started as starch is now processed as a sugar!

Mouth

Stomach

Small Intestines

Fructose

Fructose is metabolized by your liver and is likely to be converted into belly fat!

The intense sweetness of fructose triggers a dopamine release which triggers sugar addiction!

Glucose

Glucose is absorbed into your blood stream as blood sugar and is used by all cells to produce energy.

The blood sugar spike triggers a dopamine release which triggers sugar and/or carbohydrate addiction!

The Dopamine Made Me Do It

Whether it's the intense sweetness of fructose or the blood-sugar spikes from glucose, both are triggering dopamine -- the demanding "Do It Now" neurotransmitter and keeper of our body's built-in reward system.

Dopamine is responsible for our drive or desire to acquire things that give us pleasure: achievement, love, drugs, sex and yes, food.

Without it, we would lack the motivation to fuel our bodies or reproduce. Our species would cease to exist. So, to a point, dopamine is good. Until the addictive forces kick in.

The Four Ds of Dopamine

Dopamine:

1) Creates Desire

2) Delights

3) Dissipates

4) Demands another Dose

In other words, desire begets desire.

We are all potential addicts. Walking, ticking time bombs.

Here's how it works:

Dopamine relays messages from one nerve cell to the next, passing through a small space between the cells called a synapse and binding to specialized receptors in the nerve cell membrane on the other side.

A specific dopamine receptor, D2 (a.k.a. DRD2), must be activated or switched on for us to feel pleasure. Dopamine turns the D2 receptor on.

Dopamine makes us addicts and keeps us coming back for more.

Back in the caveman days, this was beneficial. Dopamine drove us towards high energy foods (like fat) and quick energy (like sugar) for our survival. It told us to overeat in preparation for winter and to reproduce to ensure the survival of our species. It told us to seek rewards as often as possible because we didn't know when they would come again.

But that's not what happens now, in our 24x7 365-day-a-year sugar-stimulated world.

Dopamine has a good memory

For some very rewarding drugs, all it takes is one "hit" to get hooked. Dopamine never lets you forget the first high.

How this works:

1) You come in contact with a cue (sight, sound, smell, or feeling).

2) A memory of past pleasure is unlocked.

3) You anticipate and expect to relive the memory.

4) Dopamine is released.

5) The drive to acquire the substance that previously delivered the reward increases.

6) You obtain the reward.

7) The dopamine dissipates.

8) You come into contact with the cue again, and the cycle repeats itself.

The more we give in to the demands of dopamine, the more sensitive we become to the cues. And, once our behavior becomes automatic, the emotional component – the desire to feel better – is no longer required. The cue triggers an automatic wanting – by-passing any attempts at willpower.

We become like heat-seeking missiles, locking onto targets that provide instant gratification. We seek things that are "new" and "exciting". We search the web. We go shopping. And we eat.

It's an itch that needs to be scratched.

The problem with this "itch", however, is that you can never truly satisfy it. You can scratch and scratch and scratch and feel momentary relief. But then it comes back.

This is the true nature of drugs – including sugar (both fructose and glucose).

It's important to note that not all addictions come from substances. They can also come from processes. And sometimes those processes LOOK on the surface, like a good thing. Take exercise, for example.

Depending on the situation, potential "drugs" include:

Substances	Behaviors
• Alcohol • Amphetamines • Caffeine • Cocaine • Food (sugar, fat and/or salt) • Hallucinogens • Inhalants • Marijuana • Nicotine • Opiates • Steroids	• Collecting/Hoarding (Shop-aholism) • Cults • Downloading music and videos • Email and Texting • Exercise • Food Behaviors (Anorexia, Bulimia, Orthorexia) • Gambling • Rage/Violence • Reading • Relationships (Other people, Co-dependency, control) • Sex • Watching the news or other television programs • Workaholism

Notice that "food" appears in both columns. Sugar Addiction as I have experienced it is a substance addiction (i.e. fructose and glucose). But food can also be a process addiction (anorexia, bulimia, orthorexia).

Also beware that many people "fix" one addiction only to have another one pop up somewhere else. For example recovered alcoholics are notorious for their new-found love of sugar and/or caffeine. This is also why it's important to acknowledge process addictions. Users may switch from a substance addiction (like sugar) to a process addiction (like shopping) and need to be mindful of signs if it becomes a problem behavior.

For an interesting overview on this topic, watch this one-hour overview on drug and alcohol addiction by Dr. Kevin McCauley:

https://www.youtube.com/watch?v=4Hz6-2NwRzE&list=FLVhLJgIqS88u srwp1LF99Yw&index=1

The on-going debate: Is sugar addictive?

There is on-going debate in the medical and scientific communities as to whether sugar and/or other foods are truly addictive.

In my experience, sugar certainly is.

And more and more research is pointing in that direction.

A Harvard study published in the American Journal of Clinical Nutrition found that sugar and other refined starches (white flour, white potatoes, white rice and pasta) produce brain activity in the pleasure or reward center of the brain, the nucleus accumbens, the same area that drug addiction affects.[3]

Researchers at Princeton have found that, like cocaine, sugar and starch stimulate some of the same regions of the brain. When these pleasure pathways are powerfully and repeatedly stimulated, the brain adapts and then it takes more of the substance to achieve the same high. Abusers continue to pursue that pleasure despite painful consequences.

In research done by Bart Hoebel, Ph.D., and Nicole Avena, Ph.D., rats preferred sweetened water to plain water. Once rats habituated themselves to drinking sugar water, they exhibited symptoms of withdrawal once it was taken away — nearly identical to those observed with other chemical dependencies — and they binged when sugar water access was restored.

Why kicking fructose can be tougher than kicking glucose

When it comes to drugs of abuse, the intensity of a drug's effect depends on how the drug is taken. The same holds true for fructose and glucose. Kicking a fructose habit is much more difficult than kicking a glucose one.

When a drug is inhaled (smoked) it reaches the brain very quickly. An injected drug also travels quickly to the brain. (That's why so many heroin addicts die of an overdose. The heroin reaches lethal levels faster than medical help can be obtained to reverse the overdose.)

Drugs taken orally enter the bloodstream more slowly than the other routes. They have to be swallowed to reach the stomach and intestine, where they are absorbed into the bloodstream. This takes time, and the body begins to metabolize them before they can act on the brain.

Fructose is most like inhalation in the speed with which it goes from taste bud to brain. Glucose is more like ingested drugs, driving up blood sugar as it is digested…more slowly and less intensely than fructose, but addictive nonetheless.

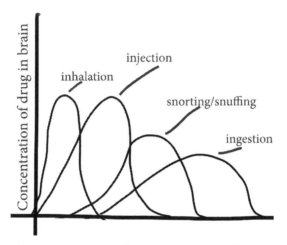

National Institute on Drug Abuse. 2006.Methamphetamine abuse and addiction. NIDA Research Report. NIH Publication No. 06-4210[4]

The Two Faces of Dopamine

Too Sensitive or Not Sensitive Enough?

Each of us is born with an individual dopamine baseline. Think of it as our pleasure threshold or what Dr. Andrew Weil calls Emotional Sea Level in his book "Spontaneous Happiness".

Too Sensitive

If you're one of the people born with a highly sensitive reward system, eating is SO pleasurable that you're likely to eat too much or too often. This is also known as the Hyper-Responsiveness Model.

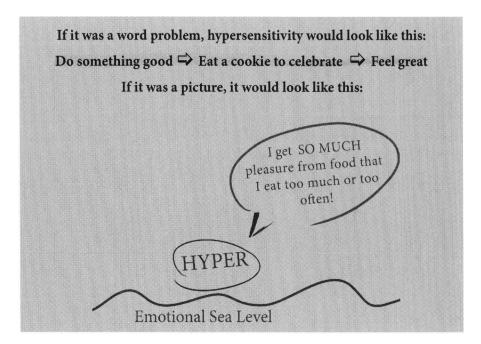

Not Sensitive Enough

Some people, including most addicts of any kind, have a Dulled Dopamine Response System (a.k.a. Reward Deficiency Syndrome or RDS).

It is believed that as many as 30 percent of us are born this way.

Dr. Kenneth Blum coined the term RDS and has done extensive research in this area.[5]

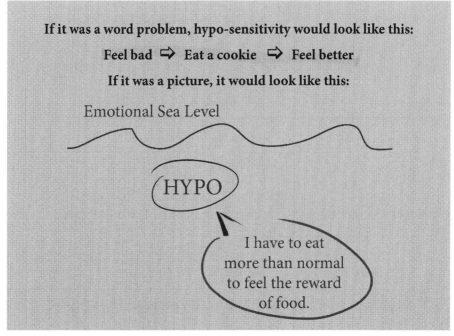

The good news is that despite being stuck with the sugar addiction low pleasure gene, you can change your brain chemistry and receptor function through food and lifestyle interventions to either improve gene expression or modify the activity, the enzymes, or the receptors, even if they are somewhat impaired.

The bad news is that whichever way your dopamine is wired, you are drawn to eat more and, as a result, gain weight.

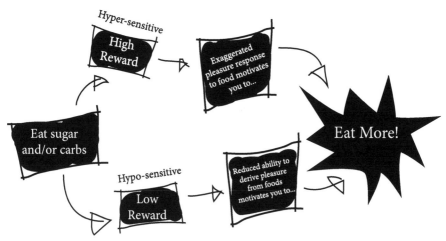

A Third Reality: Hyper, then Hypo

Some theories are that the levels change over time, and a person born with a highly responsive reward system (a.k.a. hyper) may become dulled over time (a.k.a. hypo) as they become addicted (a.k.a. the Dynamic Vulnerability Theory).

In other words:

- Are obese people obese because they have low dopamine levels?
- Or do obese people have low dopamine levels because they are obese?

Researcher Paul Kenny of the Scripps Research Institute believes that the production of and responsivity to dopamine and other endorphins may change over the course of addiction, similar to the way the body's production of and responsiveness to insulin changes as metabolic syndrome progresses — first surging and ultimately declining.[6]

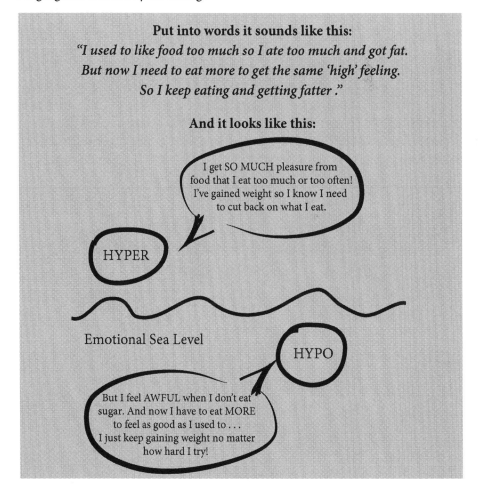

Put into words it sounds like this:
*"I used to like food too much so I ate too much and got fat.
But now I need to eat more to get the same 'high' feeling.
So I keep eating and getting fatter."*

And it looks like this:

I get SO MUCH pleasure from food that I eat too much or too often! I've gained weight so I know I need to cut back on what I eat.

HYPER

Emotional Sea Level

HYPO

But I feel AWFUL when I don't eat sugar. And now I have to eat MORE to feel as good as I used to . . . I just keep gaining weight no matter how hard I try!

The first time a drug user uses a drug, they get a high euphoric feeling when their reward system is triggered.

But neurons are smarter than we think, so when they use the drug for a second time, their cells will try everything they can to reduce the continuous dopamine transmission in the synaptic area to regulate the reward pathway.

Our brains can decrease the activation by reducing the number of dopamine receptors on the postsynaptic neuron. With fewer receptors available, a reduced signal is transmitted. Hence, we develop tolerance toward the drug and need more of the drug in the future to feel the same.

I want it…but it's not so great when I get it (a.k.a. Anticipation vs. Consumption)

Another funny thing has been noted in research.

Sugar addicts show increased brain activation in reward-related regions when anticipating highly palatable food. But they show mixed responses when they actually consume the food.

For instance, some individuals may no longer experience a great feeling of reward when consuming food, perhaps due to a decrease in certain dopamine receptors, but they may still expect to be rewarded from food, so they show activation in reward regions of the brain when anticipating food nonetheless.

So you may be driven to eat, but don't enjoy it when you do. Bummer.

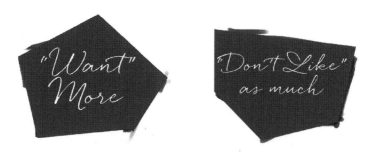

This disconnection between wanting something but not actually liking it can also be seen in the drug abuse literature, where addicts show great desire to obtain the drug of abuse, but the euphoria from taking it is not as great over time.

Digging Yourself Deeper into The Dopamine Hole

Speaking of the decreasing euphoria over time, another concept bears noting here.

I call it digging yourself deeper into the dopamine hole. It looks like putting your whole system on tilt.

Technically this refers to the allostatic state, a chronic deviation of reward thresholds.[7]

The hypothesis is that we fail to return to our baseline after using a drug. That drives further drug intake, and ultimately compulsive drug intake, and in turn exaggerates the allostatic state.

In simpler terms, the highs keep getting lower and so do the lows!

Allostasis

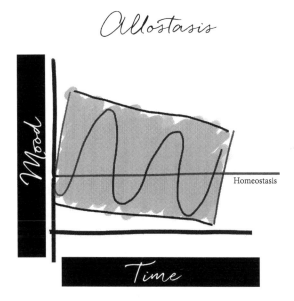

Homeostasis

The Dopamine Double Whammy:

Can you be addicted to sugar even if you can't taste it?

There's another double-whammy that dopamine packs.

It centers on the question:

- Is it the TASTE that is addictive?
- Or how sugar BEHAVES in the body?

Dr. Nicole Avena's studies have involved rats getting the taste of sugar but not the nutrient and vice versa. She has found that dopamine is released either way, which means that the two together result in a dopamine double whammy.

In another study mice that didn't have taste buds were given plain water and glucose-sweetened water. Initially they showed no preference between the two. However, after having only glucose available to them for awhile, they eventually preferred it even though they couldn't taste the sweetness.

And mice given glucose directly into their stomachs (bypassing their taste buds entirely) also got hooked on it. Dopamine levels in mice given glucose directly into their stomachs were double that of control mice, signaling the beginning of an addiction.[8]

Now take a look at our manufactured foods, like Michael Moss did in the book "Salt Sugar Fat: How the Food Giants Hooked Us." Food manufacturers have added things we might not taste (such as High Fructose Corn Syrup) to foods we don't think of as containing sugar (such as ketchup, salad dressing, baked beans, pickles, barbeque sauce, tomato paste, canned soup, cereals, stuffings, crackers and even cough medicine).

Then you wonder why you want to eat these things all the time, or why you now have a craving for donuts and barbecue wings!

It doesn't end with simple sugars (sucrose, fructose, and maltose). Simple carbohydrates and starches do the same thing, because the sweet taste is only part of the equation. After the glucose gets into your system, it's the dopamine in your brain that you want.[9]

How do I know if I'm addicted?

In my experience, foods can be addictive. Certain foods. For certain people. But you don't have to take my word for it. You can run a few simple diagnostics for yourself and see what you think.

DSM V Criteria

The American Psychiatric Association's most recent edition of the Diagnostic and Statistical Manual of Mental Disorders V (DSM V) lists 11 symptoms of addiction (technically called a "substance use disorder" or SUD).

Each of these symptoms is listed below.

A person who meets 2-3 of these criteria is considered to have a mild SUD, someone who meets 4-5 criteria is considered to have a moderate SUD, and those who meet 6 or more criteria are considered to have a severe SUD.

1)   Taking the substance in larger amounts or over a longer period than originally intended

2)   Persistent desire to cut down or regulate substance use and may report multiple unsuccessful efforts to decrease or discontinue use

3)   A great deal of time is spent obtaining, using or recovering from the effects of the substance

4)   Craving; an intense desire or urge for the drug

5)   Recurrent substance use may result in a failure to fulfill major role obligations at work, school or home

6)   Substance use is continued despite having recurrent social or interpersonal problems caused or exacerbated by the effects of the substance

7) Important social, occupational or recreational activities may be given up or reduced

8) Recurrent substance use in situations in which it is physically hazardous

9) The individual may continue substance use despite knowledge of having a persistent or recurrent physical or psychological problem that is likely to have been caused or exacerbated by the substance

10) Tolerance; requiring an increased dose of the substance to achieve the desired effect or a markedly reduced effect with the usual dose

11) Withdrawal, which occurs when blood or tissue concentrations of a substance decline in an individual who had maintained prolonged heavy use of the substance

Yale's Food Addiction Scale

Researchers from Yale's Rudd Center for Food Policy and Obesity have created a "food addiction" scale. Here are some of the questions on the scale to ask yourself:

1) I find that when I start eating certain foods, I end up eating much more than I had planned.

2) Not eating certain types of food or cutting down on certain types of food is something I worry about.

3) I spend a lot of time feeling sluggish or lethargic from overeating.

4) There have been times when I consumed certain foods so often or in such large quantities that I spent time dealing with negative feelings from overeating instead of working, spending time with my family or friends, or engaging in other important activities or recreational activities I enjoy.

5) I kept consuming the same types of food or the same amount of food even though I was having emotional and/or physical problems.

6) Over time, I have found that I need to eat more and more to get the feeling I want, such as reduced negative emotions or increased pleasure.

7) I have had withdrawal symptoms when I cut down or stopped eating certain foods (please do NOT include withdrawal symptoms caused by cutting down on caffeinated beverages such as soda pop, coffee, tea, energy drinks, etc.). For example: Developing physical symptoms, feeling agitated, or feeling anxious.

8) My behavior with respect to food and eating causes significant distress.

9) I experience significant problems in my ability to function effectively (daily routine, job/school, social activities, family activities, health difficulties) because of food and eating.

Simplified Version:
http://well.blogs.nytimes.com/2012/09/20/quiz-are-you-addicted-to-food/?_r=0

.pdf:
http://www.yaleruddcenter.org/resources/upload/docs/what/addiction/FoodAddic tionScale 09.pdf

Or my favorite, the Chocolate Chip Cookie Quiz

This, the simplest of the diagnostic tests and my favorite, is from Kathleen DesMaisons, author of "The Sugar Addict's Total Recovery Program" and one of the leading pioneers in the arena of sugar addiction.
- Imagine that you are alone.
- You come home and someone has been baking in your house.
- There is a plate of warm chocolate chip cookies on the counter.
- What kind of reaction would you have?
- Do your molecules light up at even the idea of warm chocolate chip cookies?

People who are not sugar addicts would not care about the cookies.[10]

Nature vs. Nurture:

Are your lights switched on or off?

Further complicating the understanding of sugar addiction is the fact that our physical and mental tendencies are not set in stone. Rather, they're shaped by the life we lead and the world we live in right now.

This is the concept of "epigenetics".

Science is now proving what we know intuitively—that how we live, the quality of our relationships, the food we eat, how we use our bodies, and our environment determines much about our lives.

Some people describe epigenetics like this:

"Genetics may load the gun, but environment and lifestyle habits pull the trigger."

Epigenetics looks like this:

- The light bulb is your genetics.

- The light switch is epigenetics, turning genes on and off.

Some people also call this Nature vs. Nurture.

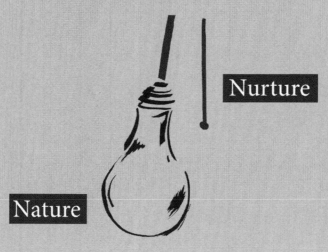

"Epi" in Greek means "above" or "beyond." Epigenetics describes how genes are turned on or off, in part through compounds that hitch on top of DNA — or else jump off it — determining whether it makes the proteins that tell our bodies what to do.

Researchers now also believe that our "epigenome" is inheritable. That means if your grandmother ate too much sugar the genetic modifications she incurred from this could affect you.

Eating Your Way to Better Genes

The role that specifically nutrients play in the ability to modify the expression of genes is referred to as nutrigenomics.

The most important thing you can do to control your genes every day is eat well. Food, and the combination and quality of macronutrients (protein, fat, carbohydrate), micronutrients (vitamins and minerals), fiber, and phytonutrients (plant-based bioactive compounds), all wash over your DNA every day turning signals from your genes on or off, up or down.

Also, depending on your genes, you may respond better to different diets— some people do better with more fat and protein and less carbs, others may not.

So what you eat matters, no matter what your initial tendencies are.

Dance of the Hunger Hormones

As if all this brain chemistry and genetics isn't enough to comprehend, now we need to talk about two important hormones that play major roles in hunger and fullness.

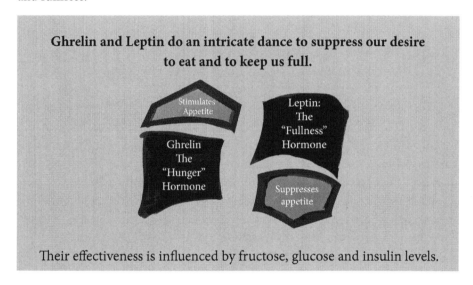

Ghrelin and Leptin do an intricate dance to suppress our desire to eat and to keep us full.

Stimulates Appetite

Leptin: The "Fullness" Hormone

Ghrelin The "Hunger" Hormone

Suppresses appetite

Their effectiveness is influenced by fructose, glucose and insulin levels.

Ghrelin: The Hunger Hormone

Ghrelin is what makes your stomach growwwwwl when you're hungry. It is high before you eat, signaling that you're hungry and stimulating your appetite. It falls after you eat, signaling that you're not hungry any more and should stop eating.

But if you're consuming lots of sweets with lots of fructose, guess what?!

Your appetite does not go down after you eat food containing fructose even though your stomach is full!

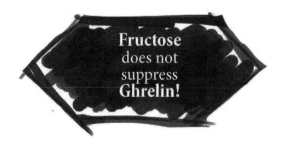

Fructose does not suppress **Ghrelin!**

Leptin: The Fullness Hormone

Leptin is released by your fat cells after you eat. It tells your brain that you're full.

It also tells your brain that you've got more energy than you need to survive so you can exercise, using up the excess energy.

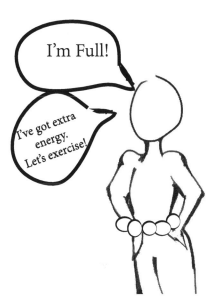

But guess what? If you've been eating lots of sugar and/or starches and have become insulin resistant, leptin is blocked from reaching your brain.

It's like leptin calls your brain, but your brain hangs up.

Your brain has become Leptin Resistant. You keep eating because your brain doesn't know that your stomach is full. This also encourages even further insulin-driven triglyceride formation, making it more likely you will gain weight.

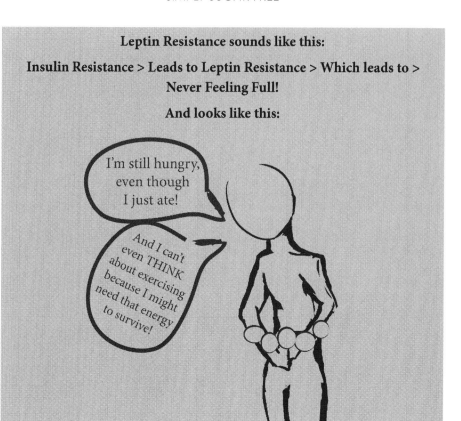

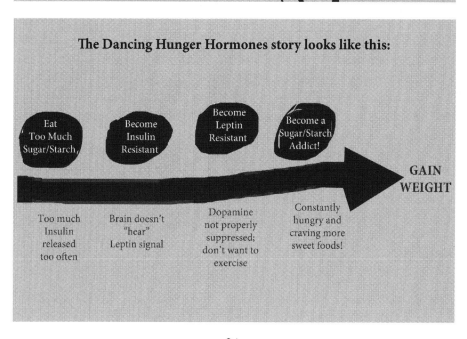

Stressed is Desserts Spelled Backwards

Now we also need to take into account the effects of stress on this complex hormonal dance within our bodies.

Our body produces cortisol when we are stressed. The cortisol mobilizes sugar from storage so our brain and muscles can work extra hard (like when we used to have to run from bears to save our lives).

Our bodies also make cortisol when blood sugar drops low and we start to feel fatigued and foggy (a kind of stress). The cortisol boosts our blood sugar so we feel clear and awake again.

> **Cortisol is a sugar-mobilizing hormone we produce:**
>
> 1) As a response to stress
>
> 2) When our blood sugar drops too low.

Some studies have shown that stress and elevated cortisol tend to cause fat deposition in the belly rather than the hips. This fat deposition has been referred to as "toxic fat" since abdominal fat deposition is strongly correlated with the development of cardiovascular disease including heart attacks and strokes.

This creates a vicious cycle: too much stress results in too much cortisol… which makes you gain weight…especially belly fat…which makes you stressed!

The New Math for living Simply Sugar Free

If you've hung in there this far, your eyes may be glazed over. But now you've got the knowledge that will help you as you begin the six simple steps of the Simply Sugar Free Process.

Let's strip out a bunch of complexity and start with:

Each one of us is unique. We have different responses to sugars and starches in our bodies and brains. We have different genetic components and were raised in our own individual ways.

So there is no "One Size Fits All" solution to Sugar Addiction.

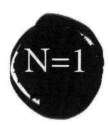

We can each conduct a controlled experiment with a sample size of one. You. Your body. And how it reacts to various food and lifestyle choices. Consider this a self-experiment that your health and happiness depends on.

Start where you are. Change one thing at a time. Track it. See how you feel. Add another change.

You may have a "flip the switch" moment when many things fall into place at once (I did). But you can also keep making small, incremental changes. Because they will add up and make a difference.

Plus, what's the downside? If you feel like crap now, fat, tired and tired of dieting, what do you have to lose?

> *The most certain way to succeed*
> *is always to try just one more time.*
>
> – Thomas A. Edison

Step into the Simply Sugar Free Process with me.

The Simply Sugar Free Process

The Simply Sugar Free Process is comprised of six simple steps designed to heal your biochemistry and change your behavior. One step at a time. In deliberate succession. Designed to help you succeed. To give up sugar for good.

You will deliberately focus on one biochemistry step until it is settled in. Then you will move over to a behavior step until that is routine. Then back to the next biochemistry step. Then on to the next behavior step. Zigzagging back and forth. Get it?

This gives time for each new step to settle in before you take the next one … focusing on either biochemistry or behavior, one at a time. Each step builds on the one before it, giving you a solid foundation before moving on to the next step.

P.S. This zigzag approach is doing another subtle thing: it's building maintenance into the process. You can see where you're going and where you've been. No falling off a wagon for you. Just hop back on to the nearest step and keep going.

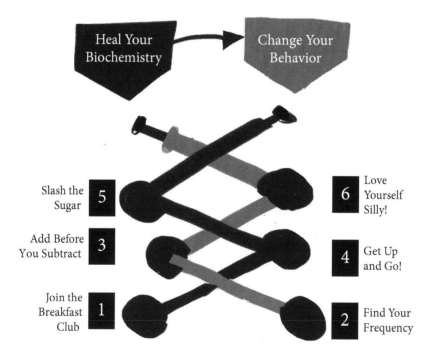

Here is a step-by-step summary of the Simply Sugar Free Process. Remember, the order is deliberate so it's best not to skip around. And remember to take your time.

WARNING: Weaning off sugar and starches will happen. But don't start there. Because if you do, you'll be right back in withdrawal hell with no net below. Bad idea. It hasn't worked before, has it?

So stick with me. One step at a time.

1) Join the Breakfast Club
Breakfast is the foundation of your day and protein is the key ingredient. Aim for at least 20 grams of protein to start the day with stable blood sugar.

2) Find Your Frequency
Develop skills to find your frequency … what works for your unique metabolism and how to balance your blood sugar and heal your brain chemistry.

3) Add Before You Subtract
Add healthy food in before taking sugar out to mitigate withdrawal symptoms and cravings. Vegetables are your new best friend. Fruit is their second cousin. Nuts can be a welcome guest.

4) Get Up and Go!
An hour a day. Do something you like. Not for the calories burned, but for the mental lift. P.S. As you get more fit, your body will reward your hard work by using more calories both during and after your workouts.

5) Slash the Sugar
Go Cold Turkey or Easy Does It. Whichever works for you. But if you've followed the steps, you'll be ready. It's not a big deal.

6) Love Yourself Silly!
Celebrate and pamper yourself. Living lean requires a steady flow of gentle pleasure-inducing activities that raise your beta-endorphins without spiking your dopamine. Recalibrate and recharge in gentle, soothing ways every day.

Living a Lean Lifestyle Forever!

The Simply Sugar Free Process takes anywhere from six weeks to six months. It's highly individual depending on whether you're a Fructose Fanatic or a Glucose Glutton (or both!), your sex (men seem to find it easier to go cold turkey), your age and your lifestyle.

But the best news is that the Simply Sugar Free Process works for BOTH recovery and maintenance.

You see, it's like tying your shoe ☺

The same process that got you off sugar will keep you off!

Maintenance is built into the process. So when you feel wobbly, down or whatever … you just run through the steps again. Where are you strong? Where have you back slid? Where can you make better choices? Tighten up your laces to give you strength?

See how the process works?

And when you're stressed or struggling sometimes you have to loosen your laces a bit. Let up until the storm passes.

But it's no big deal. If I get stressed and want to overeat, I know that if I add in extra veggies, fruit and protein I can gently guide myself through the storm without triggering cravings. When life gets back under control, I release the extra food and am right back where I was, balanced and calm. No harm done.

That's what's great about it. There's no falling off the wagon. Because there's no wagon to fall off of. As you make better choices for your individual biochemistry and behavior you are building in steps that you can rely on for the rest of your life.

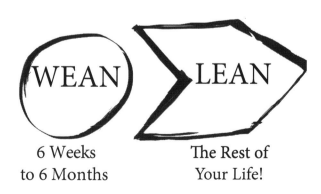

WEAN ⟩ LEAN

6 Weeks   The Rest of
to 6 Months   Your Life!

P.S. Getting Additional Support

Sugar Addiction is likely not the only issue that drives you to eat.

So just beware that you may need additional help or support, both to get off – and stay off -- sugar.

Many people find themselves addicted to food (and other substances and behaviors) as an attempt to self-medicate.

So as you go through the Simply Sugar Free Process you may find that you need additional support with other issues – the ones that caused you to self-medicate in the first place.

A Health Coach can be a good guide to help you implement these steps. A mental health professional might be needed if the issues are more severe or deeply engrained.

I offer workshops, retreats and on-line courses. Contact me if you'd like more information about upcoming offerings.

Good luck, and let's get started!

1

Step 1
Join The Breakfast Club

Breakfast and Blood Sugar 101

"I don't have time."

"I'm not hungry when I wake up."

"I don't like cereal."

"I'm allergic to eggs."

There are plenty of reasons that people skip breakfast. But there are even more reasons why you shouldn't. Especially if you're a sugar addict.

How your blood sugar works

When you wake up, you haven't eaten for hours. You're probably hungry. And your blood sugar is most likely below normal. You need to eat to "break the fast" … get it?

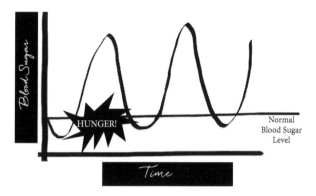

If you eat a sugar-filled breakfast (like a donut, for example) your blood sugar will spike dramatically. Then it will fall dramatically as your body releases insulin to transport the blood sugar into your cells for energy.

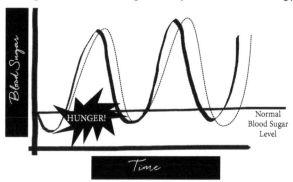

But the problem is that by the time insulin is released:

1) Your blood sugar has already peaked

2) Insulin carries away too much glucose too late

3) Your blood sugar dips too low…

4) You crave sweets and are tired, hungry & cranky!

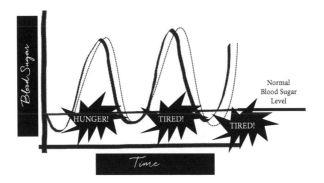

So the goal is to have a nice steady flow of blood sugar, fueled by protein, a steady release of complex carbohydrates and a little bit of healthy fat at breakfast, and all day long.

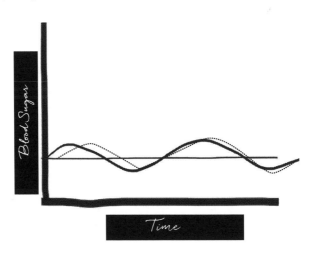

By the way, each time your blood sugar spikes the resulting insulin spike increases the likelihood that your body will store excess energy as fat.

Result: You gain weight!

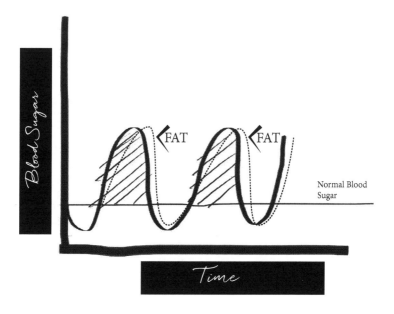

What if you're NOT hungry at breakfast?

Eat anyway!

If you're a sugar addict you might THINK that you're not hungry. But you need to eat anyway.

Think about it. Depending on what time you ate dinner and what time you woke up, it can be between six and 12 hours since you last ate. Your body needs fuel, even if your brain doesn't think so.

Here's why.

Your body thinks you might be in danger of starving and releases the pain-killing neurotransmitter beta-endorphin to protect you from the pain of starvation.

This natural pain-killer makes you feel strong and lean – you're getting a fake "high" from not eating. Beta-endorphin has approximately 80 times the analgesic potency of morphine!

Endorphins:
Your Body's Natural
Pain Killer

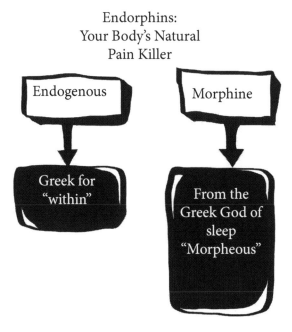

But the fake high is just hiding the fact that your blood sugar is already dangerously low and continuing to drop. If you don't eat, you will crash big time mid-morning and then scarf down the first thing in sight … and that's usually something sweet because you'll be craving like crazy and you "think" it will make you feel better faster. Wrong.

Your body also goes into hoard mode because it's afraid that no food is coming…it slows your metabolism to make your current fat last as long as possible as a fuel supply in face of famine.

So, you see, it doesn't matter what your excuse might be for not eating breakfast.

Eat it any way!

Blood-Sugar Balancing Breakfast Formula

According to the Mayo Clinic, a healthy breakfast is one that incorporates complex carbohydrates, protein and a bit of fat.

Here is what that looks like:

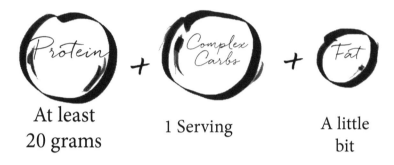

At least 20 grams + 1 Serving + A little bit

We'll get a little more detailed in the following sections ... but really, just get the big picture here.

What's a serving size?

You can use your hands to measure the right portion size:

Protein = Palm
A serving of meat, poultry or fish should be about the size of your palm. (For a man, it should be two.)

Carbs = Fist
A serving of carbs should be about the size of your fist.

Fats = Thumb
A serving of fats should be about the size of your thumb.

Fruits and Veggies = Handfuls
For fruits and veggies, grab all you can hold!

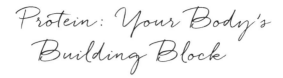

Protein: Your Body's Building Block

Proteins are the main building blocks of the body.

They're used to make muscles, tendons, organs and skin.

Proteins are also used to make enzymes, hormones, neurotransmitters and various tiny molecules that serve important functions.

Without protein, life as we know it would not be possible.

Proteins are made out of smaller molecules called amino acids, which are linked together like beads on a string,

Essential Amino Acids

Some amino acids can be produced by our body. Others must come from our diet. The ones we can't produce and must get from food are called "essential" amino acids because it's "essential" that our diet provide these.

Complete, Incomplete and Complimentary Proteins

Protein sources are divided into categories according to how many of the essential amino acids they provide:

A **complete** protein provides all of the essential amino acids. Animal-based foods such as meat, poultry, fish, milk, eggs, and cheese are complete protein sources.

An **incomplete** protein is low in one or more of the essential amino acids.

Complementary proteins are two or more incomplete proteins that provide all (or most) of the essential amino acids when they are combined.

For example, rice contains low amounts of certain essential amino acids. But these missing essential amino acids are found in dry beans. Together, these two foods can provide all the essential amino acids that your body needs.

How much protein do I need to help balance my blood sugar?

How much protein you need is controversial and depends on many factors, including how much you weigh and how active you are.

I use the formula recommended by Kathleen DesMaisons in her book "Potatoes, Not Prozac" as a starting point. At lower weights you may need a few more grams than the formula produces; at higher weights you may need a few less. Start with this formula, listen to your body and adjust as you go.

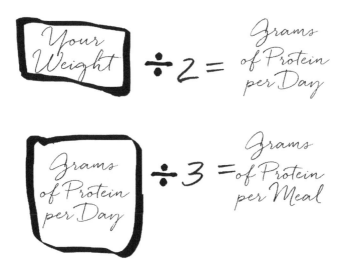

Protein content of common foods

While you're getting the hang of this new math, here is the protein content of some common foods that you are likely to choose for breakfast. If you use an on-line tracking tool (such as myfitnesspal.com) you will be able to see the protein content of all foods. After awhile, you'll get pretty comfortable with these numbers.

Food	Grams of Protein
Dairy	
Cheddar cheese, 1 oz.	7 - 8
Cottage cheese, 1 cup.	24
Egg	6
Milk, 1 cup	8
Tempeh, ½ cup	16
Yogurt (Regular), 1 cup	11
Yogurt (Greek) 1 cup	22
Poultry, Fish and Meat	
Beef, 4 oz	28
Chicken, 4 oz	40
Fish, 4 oz	24
Tuna, 6 oz can	40

Nuts and Seeds	
Almonds, 1/4 cup	8
Beans, ½ cup cooked	7 - 10
Kidney Beans, 1 cup	15
Lentils, 1 cup cooked	18
Peanuts, 1/4 cup	9
Peanut Butter, 2 T	8
Pistachios, ½ cup	6
Pumpkin Seeds, ¼ cup	9
Quinoa, 1 cup	8
Tahini, 2 T.	6

About Eggs

Most of us have gown up in the era of egg paranoia. It used to be that we believed that eating egg yolks (just the yolks, mind you) would raise our blood cholesterol and put us at risk for artery and heart disease.

But more current research has shown that this just isn't true for most of us.

You can cut the cholesterol, number of calories and fat that you get from eggs significantly by only eating egg whites. But then you will miss out on getting the choline (good for brain health!), vitamins B2, B12, D, and iron that are in the yolk.

A good option is to eat an omelet made of one whole egg and two egg whites. It's still low in cholesterol, calories and fat, but you'll get some of the important micronutrients and vitamins from the egg yolk.

What's the scoop on protein powders?

You should always try to get your protein from whole foods, such as those shown in the table. But sometimes that's just not possible.

So rather than miss your protein target, you may need to add protein powders to your foods (and often to your smoothies).

There are many different types of protein powders on the market. Here is a quick run-down of the basic types and their differences. But, as always, listen to your body. One might work better than another for you, or you might find that you need the "density" of whole foods to keep you full.

Whey

Whey protein comes from cow's milk. It is a complete protein because it contains all the essential amino acids.

Whey protein is also known to help weight loss by increasing muscle mass, accelerating metabolism and creating a sensation of fullness.

Whey does have a few disadvantages. Because it is milk protein, people with diary or lactose allergies should avoid it.

Look for whey protein isolate, not concentrate. Isolate is more than 90% protein; concentrate contains only between 30% and 85% protein. Whey concentrate also has varying amounts of lactose, which can pose a problem if you're lactose intolerant or if you have allergic reactions to lactose.

Soy

Soy is a plant-based protein that comes from soy beans. Like whey, it is considered a complete protein and contains all the essential amino acids. And, because soy is plant based, it is a great alternative to whey protein for those dealing with dairy allergies.

There are some concerns about the isoflavones found in soy. Soy intake is sometimes implicated in thyroid problems and changes in testosterone and estrogen levels. Also, some of the inhibitors found in soy have been known to obstruct digestion.

As with whey protein, look for soy protein isolate, not concentrate.

Brown Rice

While rice is mostly composed of carbohydrate, it contains a small amount of protein, which is extracted to create brown rice protein. However it's not a complete protein, so it has to be paired with other plant-based proteins like hemp or pea powder to complete the essential amino acid profile. Brown rice protein is hypo-allergic and easily digested, making it an excellent alternative for anyone with a sensitive stomach or allergies to soy or dairy.

Pea

This plant-based protein is highly digestible and has a fluffy texture. Pea protein is high in glutamic acid, which helps convert carbs into energy so they won't be stored as fat. Pea protein isn't a complete protein so it needs to be paired with other sources of protein, like brown rice or hemp.

Hemp

A near-complete plant-based protein, hemp offers the inflammation-fighting power of omega-6 essential fatty acids and is high in fiber. It's a good choice for those following a vegan diet. Some studies have also suggested hemp protein may be more helpful in weight loss, because of its high fiber content.

Complex Carbs Simplified

Complex carbs aren't all that complicated.
- Simple carbohydrates are chains of glucose that the body digests quickly.
- Complex carbohydrates are three or more chains of glucose, which take longer to process and help you feel fuller longer.

Top complex carbohydrate choices include whole grains, beans and vegetables.

Whole grains

Choices include whole wheat pasta and bread, brown rice, and whole grains like oats, quinoa, barley and bulgur.

Legumes, dried peas, and beans

The fiber in vegetables classified as legumes, such as beans and peas, helps stabilize your blood sugar and keep you full longer. They also can decrease the risk of cardiovascular disease and coronary heart disease.

Vegetables (and fruit, to a lesser degree)

Vegetables are a great low-calorie source of carbohydrates, packing in vitamins and minerals and, when eaten in their most natural form, fiber. Fruits are less beneficial due to their higher sugar content.

Some especially healthy choices are:
- Green, leafy vegetables, such as spinach, watercress, and kale
- Cruciferous vegetables, such as broccoli and cauliflower
- Citrus fruits including oranges and grapefruit
- Other fruits and vegetables with a high vitamin C content, like black currants, kiwi fruit, and red peppers

Keep the starchy vegetables like potatoes to a minimum. When you do have them, eat the skin for its fiber. Choose sweet potatoes for their vitamin A.

If the food comes in a package, use the package to your advantage

The first step toward healthy eating is to eliminate food in packages, right? But this is the real world, right?

So if you need the convenience of pre-packaged cereal or bread at least put the information on the package to good use. The information can help you make the best choice that you can to keep yourself out of blood sugar trouble.

Cereal:

- Sugar: less than 5 grams per serving
- Fiber: at least 5 grams per serving.

Bread:

- The first ingredient listed should be "whole" wheat or "whole" grain.
- If the label says "enriched" it probably contains white flour, meaning it's low in fiber and nutrition.
- Fiber: at least 3 grams per serving.

Eat The Whole Thing!

There are two main types of grain products: whole grains and refined grains.

Whole grains contain the entire grain – the bran, germ and endosperm. Examples include whole-wheat flour, oatmeal, whole cornmeal, brown rice and bulgur.

Refined grains have been milled (ground into flour or meal) which results in the bran and germ being removed. This process removes much of the B-vitamins, iron and dietary fiber. Some examples of refined grains are wheat flour, enriched bread and white rice. Most refined grains are enriched, which means that some of the B vitamins and iron are added back after processing. Fiber, however, is not added back to enriched grains.

Fiber Facts

While we're in the neighborhood of complex carbs, let's visit their cousin fiber. Fiber is kin to complex carbs because it is only found in plant-based carbohydrates.

There are two kinds of fiber: soluble and insoluble. Just like their names say, soluble is soluble in water; insoluble is not. Both are good for you, but for different reasons. Most plant-based foods, such as oatmeal and beans, contain both soluble and insoluble fiber. However, the amount of each type varies in different plant foods. To receive the greatest health benefit, eat a wide variety of high-fiber foods.

How much fiber should you eat?

25 grams of fiber every day according to the American Heart Association.

Soluble Fiber

Soluble fiber dissolves in water to form a gel-like material. The bacteria in your gut metabolize soluble fiber, and that's when the benefits start.

Soluble fiber can help lower cholesterol, blood sugar, and insulin, prevent cancer, balance hormone levels, remove excess estrogen and reduce the risk of breast cancer, make vitamins and minerals, provide food for the colon cells, and more.

Insoluble Fiber

Think of insoluble fiber as a scouring pad for your intestines. It promotes movement through your digestive system and increases stool bulk, so it can help those who struggle with constipation or irregular stools.

Soluble	Insoluble
Apples	Barley
Blueberries	Broccoli
Carrots.	Brown rice
Celery	Bulgur
Cucumbers	Cabbage
Dried beans	Carrots
Dried peas	Celery
Flaxseeds	Corn bran
Lentils	Couscous
Nuts	Cucumbers
Oat bran	Dark leafy vegetables
Oat cereal	Fruit
Oatmeal	Grapes
Oranges	Green beans
Pears	Nuts
Psyllium	Onions
Seeds	Raisins
Strawberries	Root vegetable skins
	Seeds
	Tomatoes
	Wheat bran
	Whole wheat
	Whole grains
	Zucchini

The Skinny on Fat

Remember the low-fat craze? Well, now research is showing that obesity has actually increased despite the emphasis on low–fat foods! So fat (healthy fat, that is) is not the enemy we once thought it was.

First off, fat is essential to your health because it supports a number of your body's functions. Some vitamins, for instance, must have fat to dissolve and nourish your body.

But there is a dark side to fat. Fat is high in calories and small amounts can add up quickly.

And there is concern with some types of dietary fat (and their cousin cholesterol) as they are thought to play a role in cardiovascular disease and type 2 diabetes. Dietary fat also may have a role in other diseases, including obesity and cancer.

Fat is made up of varying amounts of fatty acids. It's the type and amount of fatty acid that determines the effect of the fat on your health.

Harmful dietary fat

There are two main types of potentially harmful dietary fat — fat that is mostly saturated and fat that contains trans fat:

Saturated fat - Saturated fat comes mainly from animal sources of food, such as red meat, poultry and full-fat dairy products. Saturated fat raises total blood cholesterol levels and low-density lipoprotein (LDL) cholesterol levels, which can increase your risk of cardiovascular disease. Saturated fat may also increase your risk of Type 2 Diabetes.

Trans fat - Trans fat occurs naturally in some foods in small amounts. But most trans fats are made from oils through a food processing method called partial hydrogenation. By partially hydrogenating oils, they become easier to cook with and less likely to spoil. Research studies show that these partially hydrogenated trans fats can increase unhealthy LDL cholesterol and lower healthy HDL cholesterol. This can increase your risk of cardiovascular disease.

Both saturated fats and trans fats are solid at room temperature.

Healthier dietary fat

Unsaturated fats are the fats that provide potentially helpful dietary fat. Unsaturated fats are liquid at room temperature, such as olive oil, safflower oil, peanut oil and corn oil.

Monounsaturated fat - Studies show that eating foods rich in plant-based monounsaturated fats (MUFAs) improves blood cholesterol levels, which can decrease your risk of heart disease. Research also shows that MUFAs may benefit insulin levels and blood sugar control, which can be especially helpful if you have Type 2 Diabetes. Some good sources of MUFAs are avocado, nuts and nut butters, seeds, oils (canola, olive, peanut) and olives.

Polyunsaturated fat - Evidence shows that eating foods rich in poly-unsaturated fats (PUFAs) improves blood cholesterol levels, which can decrease your risk of heart disease. PUFAs may also help decrease the risk of type 2 diabetes. This is a type of fat found mostly in plant-based foods and oils.

Omega-3 fatty acids - One type of polyunsaturated fat is made up of mainly omega-3 fatty acids and may be especially beneficial to your heart. Omega-3, found in some types of fatty fish, appears to decrease the risk of coronary artery disease. It may also protect against irregular heartbeats and help lower blood pressure levels.

Fish high in omega-3 fatty acids include salmon, tuna, trout, mackerel, sardines and herring. Plant sources of omega-3 fatty acids include flax-seed (ground), oils (canola, flaxseed, soybean), and nuts and other seeds (walnuts, butternuts and sunflower).

30 *Simple Breakfast Ideas*

No tine? No excuses!

I get it. We're all busy. You don't have to tell me about it. I raised two kids, worked AND got a graduate degree all at the same time. But it's possible. Really. I did it. You can too!

To get the hang of combining protein, a complex carb and a little bit of fat at breakfast, here are some simple breakfast ideas to start with:

1) Applesauce with yogurt on top

2) Avocado toast with egg: Lightly toast a slice of whole-grain bread, top with smashed avocado, a sprinkling of salt and pepper, and then top with two eggs-sunny-side-up. Make it a to-go breakfast by scrambling the eggs.

3) A whole grain bagel with lox on top

4) Breakfast burrito: beef or chicken with bean burrito; or scrambled eggs with black beans, salsa and cheese

5) An egg and cheese burrito in a whole wheat tortilla

6) Beat an egg in a small bowl or coffee mug, place on high heat in the microwave for 60 seconds and add it to a toasted whole-grain English muffin. Top with a slice of cheese and a slice of tomato.

7) Cereal to-go: swap out the milk in a bowl of cereal for Greek yogurt. Add a little lemon zest, fresh berries or sliced almonds.

8) Chili and brown rice

9) Cottage cheese and strawberries

10) Cottage cheese mixed with fresh fruit and a muffin

11) Eggs, whole grain toast and an orange

12) Hard-boiled eggs, toast and sausage

13) Scrambled eggs and toast

14) Top a toasted whole-wheat English Muffin with scrambled eggs, guacamole, Swiss cheese, turkey and tomato

15) Corned beef hash and eggs with a slice of whole-grain toast

16) Oatmeal with protein powder and milk or yogurt and fruit

17) An omelet and hash browns (with the skin on)

18) A protein smoothie

19) Top plain Greek yogurt with pumpkin puree, a handful of granola and a sprinkle of cinnamon

20) Top a slice of whole grain bread with crunchy almond butter and half a sliced banana

21) A whole grain waffle or pancakes with protein powder mixed in the batter

22) Two-ingredient pancakes: Mash one banana and two eggs together. Fry.

23) A bran muffin and vanilla Greek yogurt

24) A whole grain pita sandwich with a slice of meat, cheese and an apple

25) A breakfast wrap made from a whole grain tortilla with scrambled egg, sprinkle of cheese and salsa

26) Trail mix or granola and a container of Greek yogurt

27) A multigrain bagel with a dab of cream cheese and a couple slices

of smoked salmon

28)   A smoothie made with high protein Greek yogurt

29)   A peanut butter sandwich on whole grain bread

30)   And if – and only IF – you're absolutely desperate, a protein bar
with at least 20 grams of protein. (But remember fresh, whole
foods are ALWAYS the best choice!)

And if you just can't stomach the idea of breakfast, start here

Breakfast not your thing? Ease into it with these simple steps!

1) Just add a little milk, cream or soy milk to your coffee for a small protein and carb boost to help fuel your morning.

2) As that gets easier, start to pair your cup-a-joe with a protein-rich item like string cheese, a handful of nuts, a hard boiled egg, or a small container of yogurt.

3) Once you have the hang of that, round things out with a fiber-rich, no-fuss fruit. And voila! You're eating breakfast.

PS. Don't believe me?

Read the Research

Frequently people – especially sugar addicts – don't want to eat breakfast (usually because they are enjoying the beta-endorphin induced "high" they get from not eating!).

But you don't have to take my word for it. Here's a sampling of research findings on the importance of breakfast … for many reasons.

A protein-rich breakfast reduces food cravings, prevents overeating throughout the day

Eating a healthy breakfast, especially one high in protein, increases fullness and reduces hunger throughout the day.

Brain activation in regions controlling food motivation and reward (cravings) was reduced prior to lunch time when breakfast was consumed in the morning.[11]

When you skip breakfast, your brain craves high-calorie foods

Researchers used a brain scan to look at how feeding behaviors affected the brain's "reward" center, which plays a role in pleasures and the body's response to them.

Skipping breakfast tricks your brain into thinking you want higher-calorie foods -- foods that can make you fat, or at least increase your risk for weight gain.[12]

78% of people who have maintained a 30-pound weight loss one year or longer eat breakfast every day.

Research findings from a study of people who have maintained a 30-pound weight loss one year or longer:[13]

- 78% eat breakfast every day
- 75% weigh themselves at least once a week
- 62% watch TV less than 10 hours per week
- 90% exercise, on average, about one hour a day

Eating eggs reduces hunger; decreases calorie consumption all day

Men who consumed an egg-based breakfast ate significantly fewer calories when offered an unlimited lunch buffet compared to when they ate a carbohydrate-rich bagel breakfast of equal calories.[14]

- 112 fewer calories at lunch
- 400 fewer calories in the following 24 hours

Ghrelin, the hormone that stimulates hunger, was significantly higher after the bagel breakfast

- Egg Breakfast:
    - Three eggs, 1.5 slices white toast
- Carbohydrate Breakfast:
    - Plain bagel, .5 T low-fat cream cheese, 6 oz. low-fat yogurt

Egg eaters lose 65% more weight than bagel eaters

Eating eggs for breakfast helped overweight dieters lose 65 percent more weight and feel more energetic than dieters who ate a bagel breakfast of equal calories and volume.

Further, total cholesterol, high-density lipoprotein cholesterol, low-density lipoprotein cholesterol and triglycerides did not differ between the groups.[15]

2

Step 2
Find Your Frequency

You

The Best Expert about You.

Your body wants to feel well, to be nourished, and to thrive.

If you know how to listen to it and what to listen for, it won't betray you.

But if, like me, you are a Sugar Addict, over time the addiction has co-opted your body's natural voice. The addiction is telling you what it DEMANDS. Not what is best for your overall health.

So you're going to have to learn how to find your frequency…what works for you when to balance your blood sugar, heal your brain chemistry and change behaviors to silence the voice of addiction.

Most of us have tried every diet under the sun and failed. We have piles of old food logs where we've counted calories, points and quantities for days, weeks and months.

And in the end, we failed.

So this approach is different. There is no counting. Not calories. Not points. Not quantities.

Instead you will learn how to listen to your body. What it wants. What it needs. When. To nourish you. And how to call its bluff when the addiction is talking.

I know that many people (especially former dieters) are resistant to any kind of tracking. We want to ignore our food behaviors, especially when they're bad. Admit it. As soon as you start to slip into your old eating habits, the first thing to go is the log. You don't want to come face-to-face with your failure.

But if you don't know what's going on with you – physically and emotionally – you can't find and use the critical leverage points: the gaps between what you meant to do and what the addiction made you do. And that's what this is all about.

If you develop some keen detective skills, your body just may tell you what's best for you.

Everyone needs to create a personal workbook to sort things out during the Simply Sugar Free Process. To get things out of their head and onto paper (or into a computer) so that the "data" can be sorted, filtered, analyzed and put to good use.

Just like there isn't a one-size-fits-all diet plan, there is not a one-size-fits-all way of going about making the necessary changes.

If you're a rule follower, then print out the following trackers and work-sheets, and use them religiously. If you're working with a Health Coach these trackers are a great way to share information. You can create electronic versions to email back and forth or create an on-line Google spreadsheet to share in real-time. Whatever works for you.

If you're more the intuitive type – or if you're in the LEAN phase of the process -- you may create your own way of tracking, using pictures and perhaps drawing, doodling.

Whatever you choose, try to make this fun. Otherwise you won't do it.

I like having lots of colors to doodle with as part of my figuring things out. You might want to find an on-line site or download an app to your phone. Keep trying until you find what works best for you, OK?

Remember, N+1 ... keep trying.

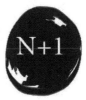

My Favorite Paper and Journals

http://www.levenger.com

I really like the high quality of all their paper products, especially with my favorite pens. I carry one of their notepads with me everywhere I go.

Their Circa Notebooks with the binding discs offer great flexibility, keeping the resulting journal thinner than a three-ring binder. I have a Circa binder that I've added to – and subtracted from – for seven years now.

I personally like a mix of digital and analog record keeping... sometimes the feeling of pen to paper adds a certain dimension to my thinking that just doesn't happen at a computer keyboard.

My Favorite Pens

http://www.pentel.com/store/color-pen

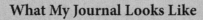

Search the web. You can find sets of up to 36 colors! Make your life a rainbow!

What My Journal Looks Like

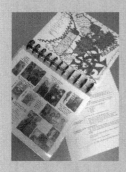

Sometimes I draw. Other times I use pictures, either as reminders or as visions for the future. Sometimes I journal electronically. I like to put my goals and some inspirational quotes at the top of each day.

P.S. I also use my journal as a Vision Board. More about that here. Follow www.hannahmarcotti.com for great inspiration. You will wish you were an artist, but it's OK if you're not!

The Mind the Gap Tracker

At the heart of slaying your Sugar Addiction is the Mind the Gap Tracker.

It's a log, of sorts. But its main purpose isn't to track what you eat and what you do to exercise.

It's more about tracking the GAP between what you plan to do and what you actually do.

Because it is in those GAPS that you can see where addiction has the upper hand.

How to use the Mind the Gap Tracker

1) Fill in the Planned Eating column of your Mind the Gap Tracker first thing in the morning or the night before.

   - As you go through the steps of the Simply Sugar Free Process you'll begin to understand what kinds of food you should eat when to balance your blood sugar and heal your brain chemistry. Those are the kinds of food that will appear in the Planned Eating column.

   - When you're recovering from Sugar Addiction, it's important to feed yourself at regular intervals. Now, these intervals might change over time as you work the process and your blood sugar and brain chemistry heal. But for starters, a good plan is to eat every three to four hours. You may need to add a snack if you get up early and lunch isn't until late. If you see that there is a long time between lunch and dinner, you may need to add a snack there, too.

2) As you go through the day, track what you actually eat and do. When you deviate from your plan fill in the Unplanned Eating column.

The gap between what you planned to eat and what you actually ate is where you will learn the most. These gaps highlight the foods, cues, habits, situations, etc. that you need to look at more closely – perhaps with the help of a Health Coach – to make sustainable changes.

The Unplanned Eating shows you where the addiction is stronger than your willpower.

Good news. Sometimes, just starting to pay attention helps us realize how often we're eating not out of hunger or pleasure but out of boredom, loneliness, frustration, or simply habit. That realization can help us deal more constructively or appropriately with these emotions and situations just as soon as we realize what's happening.

Another side benefit that might occur immediately is that when we try to eat more mindfully and consciously, we often choose foods that are better for us and start getting more enjoyment out of what we eat right away.

Mind the Gap Tracker					
		Planned Eating		**Unplanned Eating**	
		1) Fill in your plan first thing in the morning or the night before.		■ When you deviate from your plan fill it in here.	
		2) When you eat what you planned and when, check it off.			
		3) When you deviate, fill in the Unplanned Eating column instead.			
	☑	What I Ate	How I Felt	What I Ate	How I Felt
Breakfast					
Snack					
Lunch					
Snack					
Dinner					
Snack					
Activity	Note: Record your activity throughout the day as it occurs, i.e. between lunch and dinner if that's when you do it.				

Unplanned eating is what happens when:

- You walk into the kitchen to make a cup of tea. But while you wait for the water to boil, you notice brownies sitting on the counter. You eat one, then another. Then finish the pan.
- You go to the mall with your kids. You walk by the food court. Before you know it, you've got a giant cinnamon bun in your hand.
- You go into a co-worker's office to talk with her and without even thinking about it, reach for a piece of candy from the candy jar that's sitting at the corner of her desk.
- You're cleaning up from dinner and find yourself eating the extra mashed potatoes instead of putting them away.

Dangers of Unplanned Eating

- Unplanned eating is usually triggered by what you see or smell in the moment. The food that just happens to be in front of you is rarely as nutritious -- or delicious -- as meals or snacks that happen on purpose.
- Unplanned eating is usually not "mindful" – you're often focused on other things and not paying attention to what you're eating, your level of hunger, your surroundings, your enjoyment of food (or lack thereof), and how you feel after you eat. For more information about eating mindfully follow the work of Susan Albers, Psy.D., a psychologist at the Cleveland Clinic Family Health Center who specializes in eating issues, weight loss, body image concerns and mindfulness. http://eatingmindfully.com/
- It's easy to "forget" unplanned eating. But addiction has a long memory. And so does your waistline.
- Unplanned eating is rarely motivated by hunger. After all, how hungry can you be when cleaning up from dinner? You just ate!
- Unplanned eating can become invisible eating. When recalling what you've eaten over the course of the day, you're much more likely to forget or overlook things you ate without planning to. It's as if they never happened. People who do a lot of unplanned eating are often totally deluded about what and how much they actually ate.

Planning Ahead Pares Down Decisions

President Obama only wears blue or gray suits.

As he told Vanity Fair, it's a way of managing his willpower.

"I'm trying to pare down decisions," he says. "I don't want to make decisions about what I'm eating or wearing.
Because I have too many other decisions to make."

Eating all day every day requires many decisions as well. So planning ahead helps alleviate each individual decision.

Now, there are many cool, free and simple ways to track your food and activity on-line.

If you like those tools, great. They can give you a lot of important data, including the nutrient contents of your food choices.

But you're going to have trouble telling your Planned Eating from your Unplanned Eating, which is where you have the greatest chance to understand your foibles and behave differently in the future.

If you choose an on-line tool, you may want to add either a paper tracking log for Unplanned Eating or use a Google spreadsheet…whatever works for you. But the learning occurs in the gap, so be sure to Mind the Gap somewhere, somehow.

H.A.L.T.

Hungry?

Angry or Anxious?

Lonely?

Tired?

This tried and true slogan may be helpful. Sometimes the onset of anxiety or a sudden drop in mood can be traced to having forgotten to eat so our blood sugar levels are off kilter. Sometimes we may be carrying a resentment, are feeling lonely, or we are just too tired.

Asking the H.A.L.T. questions is a quick way to get in touch with your feelings and may help you diagnose what needs need to get met: food, companionship, or rest, etc.

Being too hungry, angry, lonely, or tired are conditions that leave you more vulnerable to the temptations that lead you away from recovering from Sugar Addiction. Part of recovery is learning to pay attention to these inner signals and practice appropriate ways to meet your needs.

Mind the Gap Checklist

Here are some questions to ask yourself about your Unplanned Eating:

- Where were you?
- Were you with people or alone?
- What were you doing at the time?
- What kind of mood were you in?
- How hungry were you on a scale of 1 – 10?
- How were you feeling physically (hot, tired, sick, energetic, sluggish, etc.)?
- How were you feeling emotionally (stressed, anxious, happy, etc.)?
- How much did you crave the food on a scale of 1 – 5?
- How hungry were you when you started?
- How full were you when you were done?
- How much energy did you have at the time on a scale of 1 (low) to 5 (high)?

Your brain needs glucose and sleep to make good decisions.

"Even the wisest people won't make good choices when they're not rested and their glucose is low," social psychologist Roy F. Baumeister told the New York Times. "That's why the truly wise don't restructure the company at 4 p.m. They don't make major commitments during the cocktail hour. And if a decision must be made late in the day, they know not to do it on an empty stomach."

Grocery retailers discovered this decades ago.

Researchers found that "just when shoppers are depleted after all their decisions in the aisles — with their willpower reduced, they're more likely to yield to any kind of temptation, but they're especially vulnerable to candy and soda and anything else offering a quick hit of sugar."

Completing your Mind the Gap Tracker will help you see when it is most likely that you'll be able to make your own best decisions.

It's also a good idea to jot down your planned exercise here, too, and track what you actually did. Again, with exercise as with food, you need to Mind the Gap. What gets in the way of moving every day?

Red Light | Yellow Light | Green Light Tracker

You might as well start right now to track the foods that are going to trip you up. Each of us is going to find foods that we just can't eat without wanting more.

Start that list now. It's an important piece of your detective work.

Of course you're going to find sweets on the list … after all, you are reading this book. But you're probably going to find other foods, as well.

Buttered popcorn at a movie theater is a red food for me, even though it isn't sweet. (In case you're curious, when I go to a movie I have a little bag of plain Cheerios stashed in my purse. I find the motion of eating one at a time mimics eating popcorn but doesn't trigger me.)

I also have to be careful with salty crackers and pretzels. Even though they don't contain sugar, I can struggle to stop once I start.

Red Light	Yellow Light	Green Light Tracker	
Red	Yellow	Green
Foods that I just can't stop eating once I start	Foods that I'm not sure about, but I think cause me problems	Foods that nourish me and that I like to eat

Shaping Your Recovery

Some of you will be all motivated, print out these worksheets and trackers, buy a pretty new binder to put them in and you're off. Others will struggle.

Just do what you can. One step at a time.

Psychologists call it shaping. The deal is that people are most successful at implementing and sustaining change when they make simple, small changes … one at a time.

For me, that meant tackling one meal or snack at a time.

I started with breakfast, and listened to my body.

What were the foods that I enjoyed eating just enough that I would eat them again … but never binge on them? These were Green Light Foods for me.

Then I tackled lunch. Then dinner. Then snacks. Do-able, eh?

Get Started

1) Get a journal or sign up for an on-line tracker. Myfitnesspal.com is a popular free on-line tracking tool.

2) Buy/get pencil/markers.

3) Find a dedicated spot for your workbook where you will see it and use it.

4) Write down a list of three to six physical and emotional feelings you think you feel most often onto a post-it note and stick it on the current page. You can move the post-it list to the current page each day.

5) Carry the workbook with you every day, or commit to using an on-line tracker every day.

6) Write down all the food you eat and activity that you do. But if that's too much at first, hey – just write down breakfast until you get the hang of it. Because breakfast is the most important meal of the day for Sugar Addicts. Then add on lunch, then dinner, etc. Keep "shaping" your success!

7) Don't Break the Chain. A tactic that some people use to reinforce a new behavior is called "Don't Break the Chain." This idea is attributed to the comic Jerry Seinfeld. It's actually a very simple concept. Get a calendar, and every day you track both your Planned and Unplanned Eating, you cross off the day. The goal is to do it every day, in other words don't break the chain. There are even apps for your mobile device that do this, too. For more information: http://lifehacker.com/281626/jerry-seinfelds-productivity-secret

8) For some people it's critical to track what you eat as soon as you eat it. That will make your information more accurate and reliable. We have selective memories, right? You want to know your own truth.

Here are some suggestions from the National Weight Control Registry:

Keep track of your progress. Weighing in at least once a day and keeping track of food intake is essential for most NWCR members.

Keep your diet consistent. Resisting the urge to "splurge" on holidays or weekends, NWCR members eat the same foods on a regular basis.

Show some restraint. NWCR members exert great control over their eating habits, and they rarely overeat.

Thinking about how you Think

It's no secret that we're all different. But if you understand a little bit about how you think you may increase your success at finding your frequency. Here are some different ways to look at how you learn and see the world.

Right Brain vs. Left Brain

Acknowledging whether you're predominantly right or left-brained will give you clues as to what your workbook will look like and how you can increase its effectiveness for you. (If you don't know whether you lean right or left, just Google it. There are lots of fun on-line tests and quizzes you can take.)

- Right-brain people are more creative and intuitive. They're the ones who will want markers in all 36 colors.
- Left-brain people are more organized and systematic. They'll be using spreadsheets instead.

Rules vs. Results

Another way to slice behavior tendencies is Rules vs. Results: defining the right outcomes, rather than following the right steps.

Over the years at work, for example, I've found that I work best with bosses who manage by Results, not Rules. What does that mean? That sometimes you don't need to – and don't want to! – be told exactly what to do, step by step. You don't want to be managed by the Rules.

You want to know where you're going, what you'll be held accountable for and then you'll figure out how to get there yourself (based on knowledge, skills and abilities that you already possess). You want to focus on the Results, not the Rules.

And for some of us, it just works best that way. So set up your workbook to support you in whatever way works for you.

Read more about Results vs. Rule's in Marcus Buckingham's book: "First, Break All the Rules: What the World's Greatest Managers Do Differently."

http://www.amazon.com/First-Break-All-Rules-Differently/dp/0684852861

Good Girls vs. Rebels

A third take on our different mindsets and approaches is what best-selling author Geneen Roth calls Good Girls vs. Rebels (also called Restrictors vs. Permitters) in her book "Women, Food and God."

Restrictors use food to control their life and their body. Permitters use food to numb themselves.

Roth has found that about half of us – the Restrictors – do very well on diets (at least for a while). We find rules, tips and lists comforting. We like regulations because they provide a sense of control.

Permitters, on the other hand, hate rules. They find them oppressive and suffocating. Permitters know that starting a program with rules is usually the first step toward breaking those rules and going off that program.

Both Restrictors and Permitters need to learn to listen to their bodies, according to Roth.

Since Permitters use food to numb themselves and block out their own body signals, she suggests that they begin by paying attention a few times a day to concrete physical sensations like hunger and fullness. Notice the plate of food in front of you and your body's response to it. Eat according to your physical hunger, and stop when you've had enough. Respect your body by listening to its signals.

Restrictors know when they're hungry and when they're full, but have too many rules and food facts in their heads to figure out what their body actually wants. So listen.

When you eat, just eat for greatest food pleasure!

An article in the journal Psychological Science gives us one secret to making food taste better. It isn't a new spice or ingredient.

Study participants were asked to either remember a 7-digit number or 1 digit while tasting something salty, sweet or sour. Then they rated the intensity of the flavor.

The conclusion? Multi-tasking (remembering 7 digits) = reduced taste of food.

Why? The brain has to process everything at once and the different sensory experiences compete with each other.

The multi-taskers also ate more sweet and salty foods, potentially leading to weight gain and other health issues.[10]

Transformation, not just Information

While we're making changes, let's look into a little more than food. Because what we want is a transformation … not just information.

Here are a few more things I include in my workbook.

The Daily Question

I like simple things, right? So when I heard Dr. Marshall Goldsmith speak about his "Daily Questions" practice I was mesmerized.

Could this work for me? Could it be helpful in conquering my sugar addiction? Yes!

His Daily Question Process goes like this:

Imagine a friend of yours was going to call you every night and ask you questions about your life. Write the questions that you would want that friend to ask you every day. Even the process of writing questions will help you better understand your own values and how you live or don't live them on a daily basis.

If you really have courage, recruit a friend and start asking daily questions to each other. After all, it's easier to blow off a computer than a friend! At the end of each day, enlist a friend to ask you these questions.

Each question has to be answered with a yes, no, or a number. Record the results on an Excel spreadsheet and at the end of the week you can see how well you are sticking to your objectives.

"This process forces us to confront how we actually live our values every day. We either believe that something matters or we don't. If we believe it, we can put it on the list and do it! If we really don't want to do it, we can face reality and quit kidding ourselves," Goldsmith says.

Goldsmith has been recognized as one of the top ten Most-Influential Business Thinkers in the World and has written two New York Times bestsellers, "Mojo: How to Get It, How to Keep It, How to Get It Back If You Lose It" and "What Got You Here Won't Get You There."

http://www.marshallgoldsmithlibrary.com/

Here are the questions Marshall Goldsmith has asked a friend to help him answer every day. You can use these questions as a guide to make your own list of daily questions.

I did, and found it very useful. I created an Excel spreadsheet with my own questions, printed it out and added it to my personal workbook.

How happy were you today? (1-10)

How meaningful was your day? (1-10)

How well did you plan and execute your day? (1-10)

How many minutes did you spend on meditation or positive thinking?

How many minutes did you spend on things that you cannot control?

How many minutes did you spend watching TV or 'internet surfing'?

How many angry or destructive comments did you make?

How many times did you unnecessarily try to 'prove you were right'?

How many hours did you sleep?

How many minutes did you spend walking?

How many sit-ups did you do?

How many push-ups did you do?

Did you do your strength exercises?

Did you take your vitamins?

How much do you weigh today?

Are you current on your physical, dental check-ups?

Did you pick up after yourself?

Did you say something or do something nice for someone else?

How many drinks did you have?

Did you floss?

How many minutes did you spend journaling?

The Circle of Life

The Circle of Life from the Institute for Integrative Nutrition is a visual way to measure your transformation. It helps you question your appetite for life and increase your curiosity about what you want to get out of it.

- In what ways do you substitute food for authentic fun, excitement, or satisfaction from living the good life?
- What really nourishes you and what first step is realistic for you to take to move toward that?

To complete the Circle of Life:

1) Ask yourself: What does success feel like for each area?

2) Place a dot at the center of the circle or close to the middle if you're dissatisfied in that area, and on the periphery if you're satisfied.

The new circle represents your Circle of Life.
Note: You can re-label an area to make the circle fit your life. Some ideas are:

Family/Friends
Partner/Significant Other/Romance
Health (emotional/physical/fitness/nutrition/well-being)
Fun/Recreation/Leisure
Personal Growth/Learning/Self-development

Complete this exercise monthly as you progress through the Simply Sugar Free Process to see if your circle becomes more balanced. P.S. Balance is unique to each individual – what may feel balanced for one person may feel stressful or boring for another.

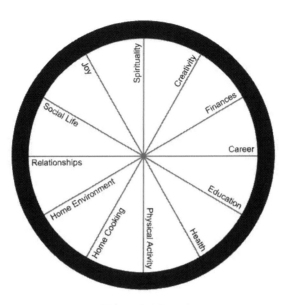

© 2011 Integrative Nutrition Inc.

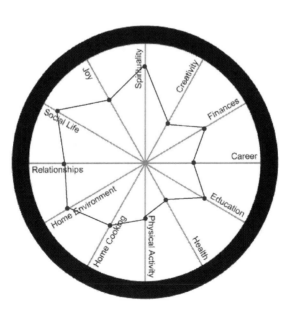

Here are some questions to ask yourself about this exercise to help you learn from it:

Are there any surprises for you?

How do you feel about your life as you look at your Circle of Life?

How do you currently spend time in these areas?

How would you like to spend time in these areas?

Which of these elements would you most like to improve?

How could you make space for these changes?

What help from others might you need?

What would make that a better circle?

What would a balanced circle look like to you?

You can also ask a good friend to complete the scores for you. An outside perspective may lead to an "aha" moment!

Add a Daily Dose of Vitamin G:
Gratitude

Each day jot down three to five things you are grateful for in your workbook. You don't need to write much. Just give each item a little thought, remembering how you FEEL when you think about them. This should take you no more than five minutes to do, according to Lorraine Miller (www.nourishbynature.com), author of the Gratitude to Bliss Journal.

There are five benefits of Vitamin G, according to the Gratitude to Bliss Journal:

1) Increased ability to handle stress.

2) Balanced hormones.

3) Enhanced moods.

4) Improved relationships.

5) Reduced cravings. When we are truly grateful for everything in our life, we have a greater appreciation for our health and the foods we eat. This gives us strength and allows us to naturally make healthy food and lifestyle choices.

Order the Gratitude to Bliss Journal
http://www.nourishbynature.com/gratitude-bliss

Download the app for your iPhone or iPad:
Gratitude Journal - From Gratitude to Bliss by Lorraine Miller
https://itunes.apple.com/us/app/gratitude-journal-from-gratitude/id793927735?mt=8

Piggyback Journaling onto Another Habit to Make it Easy To Do

Gretchen Rubin studies ways to make good habits and break bad ones. http://www.gretchenrubin.com/

One of her strategies is Pairing: Only do X when you're doing Y. (Simple but surprisingly effective.)

Connect two activities together to strengthen a habit. Sometimes, with pairing, it helps to say that one activity will occur only if the other activity occurs: "I keep my medicine by the coffee machine, and I can't make coffee until I take my pill," or "I can watch Game of Thrones only when I'm on the treadmill."

Piggyback a new habit onto a settled habit. One habit connects to the other habit. Like journaling with your first cup of coffee. Or at night with a cup of herbal tea to unwind and process the day.

Make it easy to do right and hard to do wrong.

Combine Journaling with Meditation

Both meditation and journaling create an "open-hearted space of discovery," by letting things be as they are—not changing, not critiquing, but simply observing and noting our thoughts, feelings, and sensations as they arise.

By combining meditation and journaling we can access the wisdom from the deeper layers of our being and develop a greater understanding of the messages they have to offer.

Move (five minutes). Stir up some energy: Do yoga poses, stretch, jump around, shake, make some noise—anything that lets you get in touch with your body to create a physical and emotional space conducive to meditation and journaling.

Meditate (five minutes). Once the energy is stirred, sit in a comfortable position, spine tall, eyes closed or gaze soft. Focus on the breath as you allow the energy gathered to settle and ground. Open up to your senses and welcome in all sensations.

Journal (five minutes). Express yourself from a place of spaciousness, allowing your journaling to be organic and intuitive. It could be freestyle—writing down with no direction or filter—or using a word or phrase that resonates with you (such as "without limits") as a launching pad. Write until you feel complete enough in the moment.

Meditate (five minutes). After you've completed journaling, pause, and then return to meditation. Observe the thoughts and feelings that arise from the journaling. Allow them to wash over you without judgment or attachment.

Learn from Your Journey

Now learn from your journey!
Make connections. Use these connections to refine your efforts.

1)   Review your workbook daily, weekly and/or monthly (depending on what works best for you).

2)   Review all of your Unplanned Eating. Use color pencils or markers, highlighters and Post It notes to begin to make sense of your "data".

3)   What is the connection between food and feelings? Do patterns emerge?

4)   Record the findings of your review onto a post-it note and put it on the last page you reviewed (or actually write it on that page).

5)   Choose one or more of your findings to work on as you continue through the Simply Sugar Free Process.

6)   Lather, rinse and repeat at whatever frequency works for you.

3

Step 3:
Add Before You Subtract

Eat your vegetables.

Just like your mother said. Eat your vegetables.

As many as you want. (As long as you don't drown them in cheese or butter!)

Now, we know vegetables are full of vitamins, minerals and fiber, all of which are crucial for a healthy diet. We are even learning that the more vegetables you eat, the more diseases you ward off in the future.

But for Sugar Addicts, vegetables are especially important because their fiber content (some have soluble fiber, some have insoluble fiber, and some have both!) helps balance your blood sugar. (Re-read the Fiber Facts section of The Breakfast Club for more details.)

And vegetables keep you feeling full for longer, crowding out other unhealthy eating in the meantime.

My Rule of Thumb

At least two cups of vegetables at lunch and dinner. Even breakfast, if you can (think veggie omelette or Smoothie). More if you want. But never less.

Quick Tips to add Veggies to Your Day

- Have a Green Smoothie (more vegetables than fruit!) for breakfast, lunch or a snack.
- If you don't like your vegetables plain, eat them in soups, mixed dishes and salads.
- If you make a burrito, add lots of onions, peppers and tomatoes.
- Pizza is a perfect port for broccoli, mushrooms and more.
- Add vegetables to spaghetti sauce.
- Add a handful of roasted nuts or seeds to vegetable dishes and salads for a warming crunch. Roast them first in a hot frying pan. The smell of roasted nuts or seeds is instantly comforting.

And your fruit.

In moderation.

The rule here is simple: eat less fruit than vegetables.

My Rule of Thumb

Two servings of fresh fruit a day. More if you want or need comfort. Because fruit is always a better choice than a candy bar!

Fructose in fruit isn't considered a health risk because the fructose levels are low and the fiber slows the rate of metabolism.

Five Quick Tips to Add Fruit to Your Day

1) Eat a cantaloupe (along with a protein such as Greek yogurt or cottage cheese) for breakfast, or add bananas or other fresh fruit to your cereal.

2) Have a Smoothie for breakfast, lunch or a snack. See the Recipes section for ideas or search the web.

3) Even if you're having ice cream, put strawberries or other fresh fruit on top.

4) Make a fruit salad with yogurt as a dressing. Add pumpkin or sunflower seeds for nutrients and crunch.

5) Snack on **"Fruit with a Friend."** Use this mix-and-match chart to create a healthy snack combination of your choice. The "Friends" moderate the blood-sugar rush from the fruit because they contain protein, fiber and/or healthy fat.

Fruit	Friend
• Apple	• Cheese Stick
• Pear	• Handful of Nuts
• Blueberries	• Sunflower or Pumpkin Seeds
• Strawberries	• Cottage Cheese
• Grapes	• Nut Butter (peanut, almond, cashew, sunflower seed)
• Pineapple	• Greek Yogurt
• Banana	• Protein Bar

Go Bananas!

Every once in awhile, you should just go bananas! We all need comfort food occasionally. And, although bananas are higher in sugar than many fruits, a banana is still a better choice than any highly-processed high-sugar food.

Here are 20 reasons to Go Bananas:

1) Bananas help overcome depression due to high levels of tryptophan, which is converted into serotonin -- the happy-mood brain neurotransmitter.

2) Eating a banana before a strenuous workout packs an energy punch and sustains your blood sugar.

3) Protect against muscle cramps during workouts and nighttime leg cramps by eating a banana.

4) Counteract calcium loss during urination and build strong bones by supplementing with a banana.

5) Improve your mood and reduce PMS symptoms by eating a banana, which regulates blood sugar and produces stress-relieving relaxation.

6) Bananas have a high level of vitamin B-6, which means they reduce swelling, protect against Type 2 Diabetes, aid weight loss, strengthen the nervous system, and help with the production of white blood cells.

7) Strengthen your blood and relieve anemia with the added iron from bananas.

8) High in potassium and low in salt, bananas are officially recognized by the FDA as being able to lower blood pressure and protect against heart attack and stroke.

9) Rich in pectin, bananas aid digestion and gently chelate toxins and heavy metals from the body.

10) Bananas act as a prebiotic, stimulating the growth of friendly bacteria in the bowel. They also produce digestive enzymes to assist in absorbing nutrients.

11) Constipated? The high fiber in bananas can help normalize your bowels.

12) Bananas are soothing to the digestive tract and help restore lost electrolytes after diarrhea.

13) Bananas are a natural antacid, providing relief from acid reflux, heartburn and GERD.

14) Bananas help build strong bones by increasing calcium absorption.

15) Bananas make you smarter and help with learning by making you more alert. Eat a banana before an exam to benefit from the high levels of potassium.

16) Bananas are high in antioxidants, providing free radicals and protection from chronic disease.

17) Eating a banana between meals helps stabilize blood sugar and reduce nausea from morning sickness.

18) Control blood sugar and avoid binging between meals by eating a banana.

19) Bananas contain the natural mood-enhancer tryptophan that helps to relieve Seasonal Affective Disorder (SAD).

20) Bananas make great snacks and are a delicious addition to smoothies. Add a dab of peanut butter for a little protein and healthy, satiating fat.

The Dirty Dozen and the Clean 15

Pesticides and preservatives have infiltrated almost all the food consumed in America and can be stored in your body's fat, including your brain, for years.

Each year the Environmental Working Group (http://www.ewg.org/food news/) releases its "Shopper's Guide to Pesticides in Produce." It highlights the worst offenders with its "Dirty Dozen" list and the cleanest conventional produce that is generally safe to eat even if not organic with its "Clean 15" list.

These lists help you prioritize which fruits and vegetables to buy organic, even if you are on a limited income.

Here are the best and worst of 2014:

Dirty Dozen	Clean Fifteen
Apples	Asparagus
Celery	Avocados
Cherry Tomatoes	Cabbage
Cucumbers	Cantaloupe
Grapes	Cauliflower
Nectarines	Eggplant
Peaches	Kiwi
Potatoes	Mangoes
Snap Peas (Imported)	Onions
Spinach	Papaya
Strawberries	Pineapple
Sweet Bell Peppers	Sweet Corn
Plus	Sweet Peas (Frozen)
Hot Peppers	Sweet Potatoes
Kale/Collards	

Don't like the taste? Eight days can change your mind.

We can learn to like new foods over time.

Although our food preferences are determined by multiple factors, including genes, experience and age, research has shown that repeated exposure can increase liking for a flavor in children and adults.

For example, research at the Monell Chemical Senses Center in Philadelphia has shown that people who stick to a lower-sodium diet for a period of time come to prefer lower levels of saltiness in their food.

In a separate study, infants were fed either green beans (Group 1) or green beans and then peaches (Group 2) at the same time of day for eight consecutive days.

Initially infants ate more calories from peaches than from green beans. But repeated dietary exposure to green beans, with or without peaches, resulted in greater consumption of green beans.

So eat your vegetables! You CAN learn to like them!

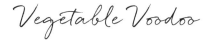

Vegetable Voodoo

There are a lot of things you can do to vegetables to add them into your life.

Roast your Brussels Sprouts (and lots of other things)

Really, I mean I REALLY like Brussels Sprouts. Even I find that hard to believe. But they have to be prepared right … not overcooked, wet and soggy but nice and crisp and browned … oozing natural sweetness. Just cut them in half, sprinkle with olive oil and sea salt, place in a single layer on a baking sheet lined with parchment paper. Roast at 400 degrees about 30 minutes, give or take. And yum! Experiment with adding balsamic vinegar and/or candied walnuts.

Slow Cook your Spaghetti Squash

Eventually, you'll want to at least experiment with taking pasta out of your diet. So Spaghetti Squash is a great add-in. You can cook it in your oven, just Google for tons of recipes. But here's a novel idea: use your crock pot! That way your crock pot serves as your butler while you're away at work. And you don't have to wrangle the rather unmanageable orb to slice it in half. Just wash the squash, poke a few holes in it so that it doesn't explode, plop it in your crock pot with 1.5 cups water, and cook 6 to 10 hours on low, depending on the girth of your squash.

Speaking of spaghetti …

When my family has spaghetti, I have "green bean" spaghetti. I just put whatever they're putting on pasta over green beans. I get fiber and nutrients … and don't feel left out!

Zip up some zucchini noodles

You can use an old-fashioned vegetable peeler or one of the new-fangled spiral slicers to come up with zoodles. Cut thin slices which you can use raw in salads or sauté. Just avoid the seeds because the seeds will make your zoodles fall apart.

Hiding Zucchini from A to Z

Just Google Zucchini Pudding and you'll find ways you never thought of to disguise zucchini in puddings and a host of other "carriers" from bread to muffins.

Sneak them in Smoothies

Nothing like a good 'old smoothie to add fruit and vegetables to your day. See the Recipes section for lots of ideas. Just remember to go heavier on the veggies than the fruits to keep the sugar content low. Aim for twice as many veggies as fruit.

Sweeten up your fries with Sweet Potatoes

Sweet potato "fries" have become quite trendy, and they're an easy upgrade to regular fries that you can make at home. Just peel and slice the sweet potatoes, drizzle with olive oil and bake at 400 degrees until done. Voila!

Cauliflower "Rice" or "Faux Mashed Potatoes"

You can easily make "rice" from cauliflower. Just cut up the cauliflower into tiny rice-size pieces, or use a food processor if you have one. Then sauté some onions in melted butter and coconut oil over medium heat until they are translucent. Add the cauliflower and any seasoning you want. Cover the skillet and cook the cauliflower for 5-10 minutes until softened.

You can also make faux mashed potatoes from cauliflower. Wash and trim a large head of cauliflower and cut up the florets and stem. Steam the cauliflower with a few cloves of garlic until it's soft, approximately 10 minutes. Drain it all. Mash or process in a food processor with some fresh cracked pepper, microplaned nutmeg and butter.

Snack it To Me!

Keep the Sugar Monster from sneaking up on you by stoking your system with healthy snacks. The best snacks have no added sugar, and combine protein and healthy fats with high–quality carbohydrates — the ideal mix to keep hunger and cravings at bay.

Most of the following suggestions are low calorie and grab-and-go.

Oranges and Almonds

For an energy-boosting bite, this snack gets an A plus. Oranges have a high water content and more soluble fiber than most fruits. Almonds deliver a nutritious package of fiber, protein, and heart-healthy unsaturated fats. Ten make a great snack-sized portion.

Want something crunchy?

Apples. Frozen grapes. Rice cakes. Popcorn. One or two large hard Bavarian pretzels. Crunchy crudités of veggies and dip (hummus, tabouli, vinaigrette, favorite dressing). Celery and peanut butter (use non-hydrogenated peanut butter). Hummus with whole grain toast. Baby carrots. Rice crackers. Nuts.

Turkey or Ham Lettuce Wraps

Want to put a fun "twist" on a low-calorie snack? Wrap two ounces of turkey or lean ham in fresh, crispy lettuce — it's a tasty combo that will satisfy your hunger and boost your energy levels.

String Cheese

One stick of part-skim string cheese is packed with protein and calcium. Pair it with an apple or whole wheat crackers and you've got your complex carbs, too. The fiber in the apple or crackers teamed up with the protein in the string cheese will keep you full.

Cottage Cheese with Nuts or Flaxseed

Cottage cheese is packed with energy-boosting lean protein. Sprinkle two tablespoons of ground flaxseed (high in omega-3s and fiber) or one tablespoon of nuts on a half cup of fat-free or 1 percent reduced-fat cottage cheese for a nutritious, filling snack.

Want something creamy?

Smoothies. Yogurt. Avocados. Rice pudding. Dips and spreads, like hummus and baba ghanoush. Puréed soups. Puddings made with silken tofu, avocado or mashed banana, mashed sweet potatoes. Coconut milk.

Peanut Butter with Celery Sticks

Peanut butter delivers appetite-satisfying protein, and it's a good source of monounsaturated (healthy) fat. Enjoy crunchy, low-calorie celery sticks with one level tablespoon of peanut butter (look for an all-natural brand with no added sugar or oils).

Pistachios

Pistachios contain the highest level of phytosterols — natural plant compounds that lower cholesterol -- of all nuts. For 100 calories you get about 25 pistachio nuts (per nut, they're the least caloric of all nuts) and, because you have to shell them, they'll slow you down!

Edamame

Edamame (green soybeans) contain fiber-rich, high quality carbohydrate, protein and heart-healthy omega-3 fats, a winning trio that helps keep blood-sugar levels steady. Buy them in the pod and steam or microwave a cup's worth, snap them open and pop 'em in your mouth — yum!

Veggies with Guacamole or Hummus

Guacamole (a heart-healthy pick, thanks to the monsaturated fats in avocado) and hummus (made from nutrient-rich, high-fiber chickpeas) both make great snacking dips. Try a quarter cup of either with sliced vegetables for your next mid-afternoon pick-me-up.

Want something sweet?

Fresh fruit. Yogurt. Apples with almond butter. Sprouted date bread with jam. Sweet vegetables such as yams, sweet potatoes, squashes cut into chunks or fries; sprinkle with cinnamon and bake. Dates stuffed with nut butter. Organic dark chocolate chips, carob chips or raw cacao nibs.

Sunflower Seeds

Sunflower seeds are high in healthy fats and protein, and low in carbs — the ideal snack ratio. They are also rich in magnesium, which may aid in blood sugar control. A half cup of shell-on sunflower seeds is a good snack portion and the shells slow you down.

Nuts

Nuts are a highly nutritious package of fiber, protein and heart-healthy un-saturated fats, plus antioxidants. Stash them in your purse or car for an emergency snack. Try one ounce (about a quarter-cup) of unsalted almonds, cashews, pecans, walnuts, peanuts, macadamia nuts or soy nuts.

Celery Sticks and Cream Cheese

Though not as high in protein as cottage cheese or peanut butter, cream cheese can be a satisfying addition to a snack of celery sticks (or another crisp veggie). Make sure to choose a reduced-fat brand and limit your portion to two tablespoons.

Make Your Own Microwavable Popcorn

Pop a bag of popcorn. Put about ¼ cup of popcorn in a regular brown paper lunch bag. Roll the top down. Microwave for 2 to 4 minutes, or just until it stops popping. While it's still hot, toss the popcorn with a half cup grated Parmesan and a good amount of chopped fresh rosemary. Or drizzle a little agave nectar over the popcorn for faux Kettle Corn.

Tuna and Triscuits

Combine a can of tuna with your favorite salsa. Use Triscuits or another whole-grain cracker of your choice for scooping.

Veggies with Cottage Cheese

Use protein-packed cottage cheese as a dipping sauce for your favorite crudités. Slice up cucumbers, baby carrots or pepper strips and pair with a half cup of nonfat or low-fat cottage cheese. You'll feel full — without any guilt — in no time!

Apple and Peanut Butter

Slice an apple and top it with a level tablespoon of natural peanut butter. High in protein, high in fiber, and plenty of taste in every bite. Peanut butter is also great with baby carrots … just don't over indulge due to its high fat content!

Rice Cake with Cheese

Top a rice cake with a slice of cheese. The cheese adds protein to keep you satisfied, and the entire snack is still pretty low in carbohydrates, making this a great choice for leveling your blood sugar.

Yogurt with Flaxseed or Nuts

Top a six-ounce container of calcium-rich yogurt with two tablespoons of ground flaxseed and you'll add a heart-healthy boost of omega-3s. For added variety, swap the flaxseed for 1 tablespoon chopped almonds, pecans or walnuts.

Want something sweet AND cold?

Freeze yogurt to make your own frozen yogurt. Make a smoothie with whatever you have in the kitchen – fruit, ice, soymilk, yogurt, carob powder. Make fruit "ice cream": peel a banana, freeze, blend in a food processor with nuts, berries or raisins and serve. Freeze a cup of grapes in a baggie for grab-and-go "grape-sicles".

Want something salty?

Olives. Pickles and pickled vegetables, such as carrot, daikon radish, beets and lotus root. Tabouli, hummus. Oysters and sardines. Steamed vegetables with tamari/shoyu or umeboshi vinegar. Tortilla chips and salsa or guacamole. Sauerkraut: will also knock out your sweet craving! Salted edamame. Small amount of organic cheese.

Hard-boiled Egg Whites

Hard-boiled egg whites give you the boost you need to keep going in between meals. Because egg whites are pure, high-quality protein, they have minimal impact on your blood sugar. Boiling eggs takes only a couple minutes; store them in the fridge to eat all week.

Turkey Rolls

Spread four slices deli turkey breast with mustard or mango chutney, wrap each turkey slice around two whole-wheat or sesame breadsticks. Or top a slice of Swiss cheese with a slice of deli turkey and a spoonful of hummus or guacamole. Wrap like a jelly roll and eat.

Frozen Berry Squares

Line an 8-inch square baking pan with foil. Sprinkle 1 c. granola on bottom of pan. BIend 2 c. fresh berries, 3 c. low-fat Greek yogurt, 1/3 c. agave nectar and 1 t. real vanilla extract. Pour over granola. Cover with foil and freeze until firm.

Warm Toasted Nuts

Toss a combination of nuts - pecans, almonds, peanuts, cashews - with chili powder, black pepper, and a pinch of cayenne. Roast in a 400 degree oven for 10 minutes until warm and toasty.

Ants on a Log

Harken back to this childhood favorite! Slather celery with smooth or chunky peanut butter. Dot with raisins.

Seasoned Edamame

Boil a few cups of frozen edamame until tender. Drain and toss with a light coating of sesame oil, red pepper flakes, and kosher salt. Popping the kernels out of the pod keeps you busy and slows you down!

Pita Sandwich

Spread the inside of a whole-wheat pita half with plenty of hummus and top with sliced tomato, onion and lettuce.

Stuffed Cherry Peppers

Stuff cherry peppers or bottled Peppadew peppers with soft goat cheese or mini balls of fresh mozzarella.

Mozzarella Skewers

Cut fresh mozzarella into 1/2-inch cubes. Skewer on toothpicks with pitted green olives and sundried tomatoes. Or with cherry tomatoes drizzled with olive oil and balsamic vinegar.

Peanut Butter and Banana Open-Faced Sandwich

Pave a slice of toasted whole-grain bread or a rice cake with peanut butter and banana slices. Top with a drizzle of honey (if you can tolerate the fructose).

Egg Salad

Get a dozen eggs and boil them at the beginning of the week. You can eat them as a filling snack or mix in some (unsweetened) mayonnaise and make an egg salad sandwich.

Stir Fry

Cook up some rice. Add your favorite vegetables and perhaps some chicken or tofu. But beware of most stir fry sauces as they're often full of high-fructose corn syrup.

Burritos

Buy some flat tortillas. Fry up some vegetables with some rice. Then melt some cheese in your tortilla and add the rice and vegetable mix. Filling and delicious!

Oatmeal

A bowl of oatmeal or oat bran is not only filling, it's good for your heart! Oats are an important source of water-soluble fiber, a potential cholesterol-lowering dietary component. Antioxidant compounds called avenanthramides also prevent white blood cells from sticking to artery walls, preventing plaque formation.

Tamari Pepitas (Pumpkin Seeds)

Toss some pumpkin seeds around in a hot pan (no oil required; the oils from the nuts are enough to keep them from sticking). As they start to sizzle and pop a little, drizzle tamari over them, stirring. Remove from heat almost immediately.

Frozen Banana Yogurt

Take a frozen banana out of the freezer. Hack it into chunks and put in a cup. Pour some yogurt over it and mush with a fork. Stick it back in the freezer. Within 5 minutes it's the most sublime frozen snack ever. Add chia seeds and cinnamon, or coconut water.

Banana Split

Cut a banana in half lengthwise. Spread with your favorite nut butter. Sprinkle with raw cacao nibs and chia seeds.

"Triple A" Snack Attack

If you're going out for a day, pack what I call my "Triple A" Snack Attack:

- An Apple
- A handful of almonds in a small bag or container
- A bottle of water (Aqua for the third "A", get it?)

Some Other Ideas ...

- Greek yogurt with a scoop of low-fat, whole grain granola.
- A handful of almonds or walnuts with a serving of dried apricots.
- A hard-boiled egg with green pepper slices or edamame.

4

Step 4
Get Up and Go!

An hour a day. Period.

I have walked an hour a day, most days, for the past seven and a half years. Walked. Not run. Walked.

I emphasize walking, because many Sugar Addicts are Couch Potatoes due to the exercise-avoiding effects of the Dance of the Hunger Hormones.

Now, if you're a marathon runner or a CrossFit afficiando, great. Walking might be too simple for you. (Unless you're using exercise as a means to eat more … bad idea!) Even then, you may be triggering stress hormones that are unknowingly hanging onto fat for dear life (keep reading for more about that).

My experience is in keeping with 10,000 of my peers, participants in the National Weight Control Registry.

Ninety-four percent of us have increased our physical activity, with the most frequently reported form of activity being walking.

National Weight Control Registry (NWCR) Findings:

-- Most (89 percent) have combined diet and exercise to achieve their successful weight loss.

-- 94% of the participants increased their physical activity.

-- Walking is the most popular form of exercise in NWCR participants.

-- 90% of the participants exercise, on average, about 1 hour per day.

-- Nearly all participants (98 percent) exercise at home.

-- 40% exercise with a friend.

Think of exercise as a savings account.

With a savings account, you make deposits, watch your money grow with interest and then reap the rewards.

You don't deposit money so you can immediately withdraw it.

Exercise is similar. It also gathers interest: As you get more fit, your body rewards your hard work by using more calories during and after your workouts.

> Going for a walk for an hour is one hour you don't spend sitting in a chair or on your couch – significant because prolonged sitting is associated with increased risk of diabetes and overall mortality.

Exercise is so much more than just burning calories. The calories burned during exercise, unless you're a professional athlete, make up a small portion of the calories you burn in a day; what you eat has a much greater influence on your body weight.

So why should we bother to exercise? Because burning a few calories is just the tip of the iceberg – exercise is an indispensible component of a healthy lifestyle, and has profound beneficial effects, especially on the heart and brain.

- Muscle burns calories while fat does not.
- A pound of muscle takes up less room than a pound of fat.
- Exercise builds muscle, which increases your body's resting metabolic rate, so you expend more calories even when you're not exercising.
- Exercise helps maintain muscle.
- Because muscle burns calories, exercise can also help you maintain the weight you lose, which is often harder than losing weight.

Researchers estimate that your body continues to burn calories at a higher rate for between 2 and 24 hours after you finish exercising.

If you have not exercised in a while or plan to do more than walking, check with your physician prior to starting to exercise. Moderate-intensity aerobic activity, like brisk walking, is generally safe for most people.

More is not necessarily better if you go beyond the right "zone" for your body. The key is to get the right mix for your needs. No easy answers, no one-size-fits-all solutions. This, once again, is a task for you to sort out what is right for you.

P.S. The rule of thumb is to walk 14,000 steps a day to lose weight; 10,000 steps a day (about five miles) to maintain.

What if your "Get up and Go" got up and went?

The good news is that the motivation to get up and go is a circular process.

- The less fit you are, the less likely you are to exercise. The less exercise you do, the more your fitness level drops. Round and round and you get rounder.

- But the cycle works in reverse as well. The fitter you become, the more you will want to exercise and the more fit you will become.

And take heart, the worse you are to begin with, the more dramatic the results will be.

> **"Movement in your body means movement in your life."**

People who love running or lifting weights find these types of activities highly rewarding, because their dopamine is working for them.

Obese people often have abnormalities in brain dopamine activity that could help explain why they are less likely to engage in voluntary physical activity and/or need a greater stimulus to get the same feeling as someone with normal dopamine functioning.[16]

In one study of obesity, individuals with the lowest number of dopamine receptors (D2) had the largest BMI. Because dopamine modulates motivation and reward circuits, a dopamine deficiency in obese individuals may perpetuate over-eating to compensate for decreased activation of their motivation and reward circuits.[17]

But the question still arises:

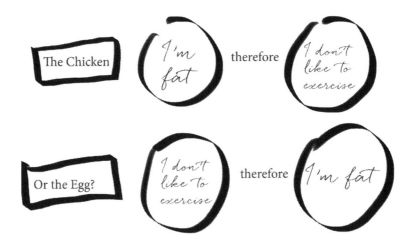

The answer may be that this depends, over time.

And can be changed through healthy nutrition and lifestyle choices.

Put one foot in front of the other.

It's a simple as that.

Walking, especially slow leisurely walking, does more than burn calories.

Only a few lifestyle choices have as large an impact on your health as physical activity. People who are physically active for about 7 hours a week have a 40 percent lower risk of dying early than those who are active for less than 30 minutes a week.

What Makes Walking Different than Other Types of Exercise

- Walking is one of the only forms of exercise that lowers, rather than raises, stress hormones. Feel like your stress is the reason you're having blood sugar issues and craving sweets? Walk!
- Walking is one of the only forms of activity that reduces rather than increases hunger. And because of its effect on stress hormones, it may even reduce cravings as well.
- Leisurely walking is one of the only forms of exercise you can do as much as you like with little concern for over-training.

Emotional Benefits of Walking

- Walking obviously has an impact on your physique and stamina. But it also has many important emotional benefits.
- Walking distracts you from your problems. A change of scenery while walking can take your thoughts away from stressful issues. Choose a route that is enjoyable visually and vary it for variety.
- Walking improves your ability to solve problems. When you walk, you think. Walking expands mental productivity. As you reflect on different scenarios, answers come. Walking can ease the struggle of decision making, allowing you to come to a solution in a less stressful manner.
- Walking boosts your creativity. When you walk, you think. New ideas emerge as you let your imagination do its thing. Inspirations can come from a walk that will surprise you. Be expectant.

- Walking enhances your social network. Whether you invite a friend to join you or simply enjoy the opportunity of spontaneous conversations with others you encounter, walking and talking go together. Meshing the two together is an obvious match.
- Walking helps you feel better about yourself. When finished with a walk, the sense of accomplishment you feel about exercising will contribute to your self-esteem and increase your motivation to do it again the next day.
- Seems kind of odd the simple act of walking can either distract from or help to solve problems, but it does. Use walking for either approach, whatever makes most sense at the time. Walking improves your emotional state giving you an additional tool to cope with stress.

50 Reasons Walking is Good for You

If you still need convincing, here are 50 reasons why walking is good for you.

1) Almost everyone can do it.

2) It doesn't require special equipment.

3) It is one of the easiest ways to get more active.

4) It reduces symptoms of depression and anxiety.

5) It is a low impact exercise.

6) Walking makes the heart work smarter, not harder.

7) It lowers low-density lipoprotein (LDL) cholesterol, the "bad" cholesterol.

8) It raises high-density lipoprotein (HDL) cholesterol, the "good" cholesterol.

9) It lowers blood pressure.

10) It reduces the risk of some cancers.

11) In older adults, regular walking has been shown to decrease the risk of cognitive impairment and contribute to maintenance of brain volume.

12) It helps reduce the risk of Type 2 Diabetes.

13) It helps manage Type 2 Diabetes.

14) It improves mood.

15) It helps maintain strong muscles and bones.

16) It reduces the risk of heart attack.

17) It is less likely to lead to injuries than many other forms of exercise.

18) It reduces the risk of heart disease.

19) You don't have to pay for it.

20) It builds aerobic fitness.

21) Walking affects the levels of several neurotransmitters in the brain, including increasing the production of serotonin, which is associated with feelings of well-being.

22) It helps maintain lean muscle tissue.

23) Walking protects against osteoporosis, because it increases muscle strength and muscle strength is the best predictor of bone strength.

24) You can do it almost anytime, anywhere.

25) Exercise helps to bring the human mind into the present moment, becoming intensely aware of sensations in the body, rather than day-dreaming. A study published in Science found that the human mind is daydreaming (not thinking about its current task) about 47% of the time, and also that people rated their mood as happier when they were focused on their present activity rather than engaging in other thoughts.

26) You can do it outdoors and benefit from nature.

27) You can listen to music while you walk, further increasing the pleasant effects.

28) You can do it alone, or with friends.

29) Staying physically active is far more likely to determine a woman's future risk of heart disease than any other well-known factor, including

smoking, obesity and high blood pressure. University of Queensland researchers found that physical inactivity served as the leading risk factor for heart disease at every age from the early 30s to late 80s of more than 32,000 Australian women.

30) Walking makes your brain happy. It is nature's mood elevator.

31) You don't have to go to a gym filled with young, vigorous, shapely people strutting around with gorgeous bodies that you will invariably feel you need to compete with.

32) It can improve your ability to do daily activities and prevent falls, if you're an older adult.

33) It increases your chances of living longer.

34) It reduces your risk of developing metabolic syndrome, a condition in which you have some combination of too much fat around the waist, high blood pressure, low HDL cholesterol, high triglycerides, or high blood sugar.

35) Walking can improve your quality of life if you are a cancer survivor.

36) Doing aerobic, muscle-strengthening and bone-strengthening physical activity of at least a moderately-intense level can slow the loss of bone density that comes with age.

37) It helps with arthritis and other conditions affecting the joints.

38) It can help keep your thinking, learning and judgment skills sharp as you age.

39) It can reduce your risk of depression and may help you sleep better.

40) It can help reduce your risk of falling as you age.

41) It can enhance self-esteem.

42) It combats depression.

43) It triggers the release of endorphins, potent brain chemicals that relieve pain and stimulate relaxation. Simply put, the higher your level of endorphins, the greater your sense of calm and well-being. No wonder walking can make you feel so good.

44) It can be especially effective for women who have postpartum depression.

45) It can help reverse sarcopenia, a condition associated with inactivity and aging in which fat replaces muscle. According to one study, postmenopausal women were able to reverse muscle-mass loss after two months of small increases in physical activity and strength training. This was linked to better overall health, better balance and fewer falls.

46) Walking builds our antioxidant defenses.

47) Walking enhances sleep.

48) Walking protects against chronic inflammation.

49) You will discover the miracle of time expanding. Exercise and you will have more focused energy than you ever dreamed of.

50) If you exercise regularly, you will get better at it and start to like it. At first, it may feel cumbersome and very uncomfortable, but over time exercise will become enjoyable. Eventually, it becomes so routine and so enjoyable that if you don't exercise for a few days, you will miss it terribly. (Really. I promise.)

So…what are you waiting for? Get up and Go! Your body and mind will thank you.

Into the Woods

While walking anywhere can act to balance the nervous system and make us feel more relaxed, walking in a nature setting like the woods seems to have an even greater impact.

A study out of Japan published in the Journal of Physiological Anthropology in March of 2007 showed some very interesting metabolic effects of walking especially when done in a natural environment.

In this study researchers examined the impact of walking in different environments on cortisol levels, immune responses and nervous system balance. Twelve subjects were recruited for the study and had physiological measures of stress taken six times during the day. Once in the morning on waking, before and after a 15 minute walk either in the woods or the city, before and after watching scenery of the woods or the city on a television, and once in the evening before bed.

The measures taken were heart rate variability (a sensitive measure of stress balance in the body assessed through looking at the heart), blood pressure, pulse rate, salivary cortisol (the best measure for cortisol levels), and secretory IgA (a measure of immune activity). In addition, subjective measures of comfort, calm and feelings of relaxation were also assessed.

The researchers showed a significant lowering of cortisol levels from walking in the woods versus walking in the city despite an equal amount of time spent walking in each setting. In addition, both systolic and diastolic blood pressure readings were significantly lower before, during and after walking in the woods vs. walking in the city. Heart rate variability (HRV) was also higher walking in the woods indicating a shift toward the parasympathetic (relaxing) side of the nervous system.

Not surprisingly, subjective feelings of relaxation, comfort, and calm were also enhanced in the woods vs. the city. Similar patterns were observed when the subjects watched the scenery on a TV vs. actually walking it. This indicates that something about the nature scenery was having a strong impact.

This study shows that exercise is not always just about calories, but that the hormonal activity generated in response to the surrounding environment is also having an impact.

A lower cortisol level along with lower perceived feelings of stress will have a positive impact on fat loss both directly, through less cortisol activity, but also indirectly through potential decreases in hunger and cravings for sweets or fatty foods which cortisol will impact.

Getting the right fuel(s) for Exercise

Our bodies use two types of fuel to drive our muscles, carbohydrates and fat.

Like a car that can run on either gas or electricity, we too have more than one way we can power our machine.

And ultimately, there are two places we can get that fat and sugar from:

1) The fat and sugar in our diet.

2) The fat and sugar stored in our bodies.

In other words, we can use the food we just ate – either the fat or sugar in it – as a source of fuel. Or we can use stored forms of fat and sugar in the body.

Our bodies were designed to store fat because fat is the best and most efficient fuel. You were originally designed as a fat BURNING machine (not a fat storing machine).

Long ago, you ate what you caught or gathered. Food came at infrequent or unanticipated intervals. When rabbits and roots were available, you ate them. When they weren't, you depended on your fat stores. Getting fat was not an issue.

You burned what you stored and you used what you ate.

For Sugar Addicts, our bodies generally burn sugar because that is most of what we give them (sugar and white things). And because we've given our bodies a glut of sugar, the sugar satisfies the little bit of exercise we are most likely to do. We never get to the fat burning stage.

We need to help our bodies remember how to burn fat. Exercise does that.

Don't exercise on Empty

Make sure to plan your meals, snacks and exercise to avoid exercising on empty.

To boost your stamina, eat a 150 to 200-calorie snack that contains one to two servings of carbohydrates about 30 minutes to 1 hour before exercise.

Here are some examples. Many of the *Snack it to Me* examples in *Step 3: Add Before You Subtract* are useful, too.

- An apple with 1 tablespoon of peanut butter or a handful of mixed nuts
- One ounce of string cheese and 6 crackers
- A protein bar with about 150 calories and at least 10 grams of protein.

Eat less, exercise more:

Equation for an Epic Fail!

Eat less, exercise more to lose weight is what we have been told for years. But it is the equation for an epic fail. You'll just be hungry and tired all the time. The new weight loss equation is one that is tailored to your own specific biochemistry.

The best option is a new equation which says:

1) Eat the right amount of the right foods at the right time for your body.

2) Exercise at the right level of intensity to get the results you want.

Less can be more

Strenuous exercise triggers the stress-fighting hormone cortisol, which drives sugar into the blood to deliver a life-saving burst of energy. It also temporarily suppresses hunger but shortly thereafter it triggers a hunger for calorie-rich comfort foods.

This hunger is in part due to a cortisol-induced insulin response. During strenuous exercise, insulin drives sugar into the muscles to fuel the exercise or, as the body may perceive it, whatever emergency is at hand.

After exercise, cortisol and insulin surge to refuel your body, leaving you hungry.

Excess Fuel Packs around the Middle

Insulin and cortisol both have an affinity for storing any unused fuel or sugar as visceral or belly fat, rather than as subcutaneous fat elsewhere in the body. In fact, when it comes to cortisol and insulin surges, the body is four times more likely to store fat around the belly than anywhere else in the body!

The Hormonal Hunger Response

Heightened stress levels that stimulate cortisol and insulin inhibit the production of leptin (the appetite hormone that tells you when you are full).

Stress also stimulates the production of the "huger hormone" ghrelin. Both of these hormonal effects stimulate hunger as a result of perceived stress by the body. (The Hunger Hormones dance again.)

In other words, if you were to exercise long or hard to get the body to burn stored fat as fuel, you would have to figure out how to resist the very strong hormonal impulse to eat fat-storing, calorie-rich comfort foods that follows shortly after the workout.

So less can be more.

15 Ways To Sneak Exercise into your day

Walking for an hour is a great choice. But here are 15 other ways to sneak exercise into your day.

1) Gardening

2) Dancing (Ballroom, Line Dancing, Square Dancing)

3) Walking your dog

4) Doing yoga

5) Playing basketball

6) Bowling

7) Fishing

8) Raking Leaves

9) Swimming Laps. "Swimming is the ultimate form of sensory deprivation," Diana Nyad has said. "You are left alone with your thoughts in a much more severe way."

10) Hiking

11) Lifting Weights

12) Wii Boxing

13) Walk or cycle to work (or your local bus or rail station, if you're a commuter). Simply wear athletic shoes and keep an extra pair of dress shoes at the office. Or bring a pair of athletic shoes to work and fit in a walk on the way home. Weather permitting.

14) If you work at home break up your day with a workout break. Instead of taking a 20-minute break to read the paper and have a snack, stretch the break out a few minutes longer and enjoy a long walk, bicycle ride (outdoors or on a stationary bicycle in bad weather) or swim, or watch a favorite aerobics DVD. An exercise break is even more relaxing than putting your feet up.

15) Lunchtime can be a good time for a walk, cycle or swim. If you're a swimmer or prefer going to a health club, your pool or club should be close to where you work or live.

20 Ways To Make Moving Fun

If exercise isn't fun, you won't do it. So here are 20 ways to make moving fun.

1) Start with short, easy walks. Increase the length and/or intensity from there. But don't increase both at once!

2) Be sure your shoes fit well. Before wearing them during a long walk or workout, spend time breaking them in by walking around in them for short periods of time.

3) Don't exercise to eat, eat to exercise. Food is fuel, not the enemy. Don't over-exercise just so you can eat more.

4) Know what you like. The best exercise for you is one that you like. If you're doing something that you hate, you're not going to keep doing it.

5) Know your intensity. Some people love high intensity workouts like CrossFit or running. Personally, running makes me anxious. I prefer to walk. That is sustainable for me.

6) Have a workout buddy. Everyone has their off days. Whether it's a lack of motivation or a compulsion to overdo it, one of the most effective safety nets is having a workout buddy.

7) Do it on your terms. Along with finding a fitness plan you enjoy, work out when and where you like.

8) Mix things up. Balance walking with a mixture of activities, such as cardio and strength training, or arm days and leg days.

9) Do it for the mental benefits. Exercise is an effective coping method for stress, anxiety and depression, and healthy exercisers harness these powers for good.

10) Be flexible on scheduling. Scheduling exercise into your day like you would any other appointment can help you stick with your fitness plan. But you also need to be flexible. Some days a regular workout just gets bumped from the schedule. When that happens, keep things in perspective. Try to be active in other ways without losing sleep over it. It happens.

11) Know when to say when. You want to feel like you worked hard and you want some fatigue. But feeling so exhausted that you just want to drop at the end of the day is not the goal!

12) The number one reason given for not exercising is lack of time. That's why it is important to include exercise in your Mind the Gap Tracker. Plans can change — but it's best to have a plan, even if you have to change it. Tracking Planned and Unplanned exercise will help you see if and why you tend to skip scheduled exercise.

13) Your own schedule might involve a variety of workout times — morning workouts on some days, for example, and lunchtime or after-work exercise sessions on other days. The key is to find a blend that works for you and to stick with it. Use your Mind the Gap Tracker to schedule your planned workouts in advance. Check off each workout when you're finished and even make notes for yourself.

14) Turn family activities into opportunities to move. If you're planning to go to a beach or park, take an invigorating walk on the beach or a bike ride through the park.

15) You don't need to get all your exercise in one session. If you're aiming for an hour of exercise each day, you can split it up over two half-hour sessions (for example, at lunchtime and again after work).

16) Many gyms have TVs and personalized radio stations on stationary bikes and treadmills.

17) If you work out at a health club bring your own earphones. Most have TVs set up so that you can watch whatever channel is most interesting. Finding a television show can make 30 minutes fly by.

18) Shape up your arms while you walk. Use soup cans as weights for your arm exercises.

19) Put your stationary bicycle in front of a TV, or get a book holder for your iPad or laptop. Time passes much more quickly when you're entertained!

20) Find your favorite tunes, put them on your iPod or music player and rock out while you walk out! Choose a mixture of fast beat and slow beat music. Then walk to the beat of the music that is playing. Create a playlist for the length of time you are going to walk. Then your walk becomes a matter of songs, not miles or minutes.

Move and Meditate, all at once

I'm all for multi-tasking and efficiency if I can get more done in less time. So one of my favorite "life hacks" is to move and meditate, all at once.

Uniting three rhythms -- stepping, breathing and mental counting -- is one of the most effective ways to calm and redirect a chattering mind

Pick a safe and quiet place to walk, such as a park or a local school track, where you have room to wander.

Then try this technique.

1) Start by standing still and taking a moment to get in touch with your physical body. Stand and notice your body and how it feels.

- Notice the weather around you.
- Relax your face. Let any tension in your scalp or jaws dissipate.
- Let your shoulders relax and let your arms hang naturally.
- Take a few deep breaths right down into your stomach and feel all the muscles in your torso relax as you exhale.

2) Begin walking at a normal pace, with your arms relaxed at your sides or with your hands together at your navel.

- The repetitive movement of your legs and feet is like a physical mantra, rather than a mantra that you repeat to yourself mentally. The key is to absorb yourself in this rhythmic sensation, and to let go of any thoughts if they arise.
- Try synchronizing your thoughts or your breathing with your walking pace. For example, you can repeat a mantra mentally in time with your steps, or you may choose to count your steps as you walk. Try synchronizing your breath slowly and deeply in time with your steps, breathing in for four steps and then breathing out for four steps.
- You can also walk in time to meditation music. This type of music contains a repeating foundation of mantra-like notes that help to still your mind.
- Devote your attention to your body and its movement. Return your attention back to that movement whenever your mind wanders off.

3) Go as far as you can until you come to a fence or other boundary, then slowly stop, turn around and walk back the same way to where you started.

4) Lastly, come to a natural stop and just experience yourself standing. Notice what it's like to no longer be mobile. Simply stand, and experience yourself.

P.S. It's OK for you to look around during this meditation. After all, you need to be aware of your surroundings to some degree so that you don't trip over anything along the way.

Leisure Walking + Meditation = Stress Reducing Effect of Brisk Walking

For the study, researchers recruited 135 volunteers and divided them into five groups. Three of the groups took up walking—one at a brisk pace, the other two at a low-intensity pace. The fourth group practiced mindful exercise, which is based on the principles and movements of Tai chi. The fifth group served as controls—meaning they were asked not to change anything about their lives.

In addition, one of the groups assigned to walk at a low-intensity pace learned a simple meditation technique to practice while exercising. All they had to do was pay attention to their footsteps, counting "one, two, one, two" and visualizing each number in their minds as they went along. If they found their thoughts drifting to other matters, they simply said, "Oh, well" and resumed counting their footsteps.

The combination of meditating and low-intensity walking produced dramatic results, according to cardiologist James Rippe, MD, in the Nov. 2011 issue of Prevention Magazine (http://www.prevention.com/fitness/fitness-tips/reduce-stress-walking-exercise).

During the 16 weeks of the study, the people who meditated while they walked reported decreases in anxiety, along with fewer negative and more positive feelings about themselves. In fact, the benefits were equal to those associated with brisk walking. Even better, they were evident after just one session, and they lasted for the duration of the study.

By comparison, the people who walked at a low-intensity pace but didn't meditate showed no improvements until the 14th week, and even then, the effects weren't as significant.

On the other hand, the people who engaged in mindful exercise experienced results that were very similar to those reported by the walking-plus-meditation group, suggesting that other mental techniques could yield stress-busting benefits.

According to Rippe, one of the most impressive findings from this research is the immediacy with which walking can relieve stress.

The study also provided good news for those who aren't able to engage in high-intensity exercise: They can capitalize on walking's stress-busting effects just by practicing meditation or another mental technique during their strolls.

And for those who find relaxation exercises tedious or boring, the study proved that a brisk walk can do just as good a job of short-circuiting stress.

Add Nasal Breathing to further reduce stress

Dr. John Douillard in his book "Body, Mind and Sport" advocates a "less is more" approach to working out using Nasal Breathing. At a retreat at the Omega Institute, I participated in this practice with Dr. Douillard himself.

Breathing through the nose while walking is a tool that can alter the body's perception of an activity it might normally perceive as stressful, to one of calm and repair. Proper nasal breathing allows the body to respond to exercise without the fat storing, hunger provoking response.

Douillard calls this effect the eye of the hurricane. It's the ability to be calm in the midst of dynamic activity. The bigger the eye of the hurricane, the more powerful the winds – the calmer we are, the more effective and powerful we can be.

- Keep your mouth closed, and breathe in and out through your nose while you walk. Count your steps as you do.

- As you inhale, allow your entire rib cage to expand by pulling the air deep into the lungs where there is a higher concentration of oxygenated blood and calming nerve receptors. Breathing into the more oxygen-rich lower lobes of the lungs and activating a calm nervous system response to exercise wards off the release of stress response hormones.
- As you exhale, contract your rib cage completely to force all of the air out of your lungs.
- This type of breathing induces a relaxation response by stimulating the nerve receptors in the lower lobes of your lungs. Read more about its benefits here: http://lifespa.com/15-benefits-nose-breathing-exercise/

25 Ways To Work Out @ Work

What's your solution to the mid-afternoon blahs when you're fresh out of ideas and energy and work is piled up on your desk? Caffeine? Sugar? Please, no!

Part of the problem of that daily slump is too much sitting. Just getting up and strolling around the office could rev you up for the rest of the workday. Research tells us that if you need inspiration, fresh ideas or even the mental energy to complete the work on your desk, the answer is exercise. Or shall we call it desk-ercise?

Moving your body benefits your brain. The secret is the blood flow exercise generates – it goes to your head where it can nourish a protein called brain-derived neurotrophic factor (BNDF for short) that gets those neurons in gear so that you're better able to problem solve, strategize and absorb new information.

Research suggests that you can get this brain boost with only 20 minutes of aerobic exercise at 60 to 70 percent of your maximum heart rate. (To calculate that subtract your age from 220 and then multiply by .60 to .70.)

1) Sit in a chair and alternatively raise your left and right knee toward your chest, five times each.

2) Try using a balance ball instead of a chair for increased core strength.

3) Get up from your desk at least once an hour.

4) Try the neck stretch: Touch your ear to your shoulder and hold it there. Repeat on the other side.

5) For a chest opener, stretch your arms back as if you were trying to grab a pencil between your shoulder blades.

6) Stand in a doorway, hold the door frame on each side and walk forward until you feel a stretch in your chest.

7) Keep a rebounder nearby or in a break room for a quick "bounce'" of energy.

8) Try supported back extensions. Hold your hips and gently extend your back by bending backward.

9) Stand in front of a small trashcan and lift up those legs to tap your toes on its edge, alternating feet, like a soccer drill.

10) Try the "Wooden Leg." Sit in your chair. Extend one leg out straight in front of you. Hold for two seconds. Then raise it up as high as you can, and hold it again for two seconds. Repeat with each leg 15 times.

11) Take the stairs (two at a time!), not the elevator.

12) Instead of slogging away for hours nonstop, take a mini break for a stationary jog. Pop up from your chair and jog in place. Pick up your knees to increase the effort.

13) Get up from your desk and go talk to your co-workers instead of e-mailing them.

14) Try the Namaste: Seated upright with feet flat on the floor, bring your palms together in front of your chest and push both hands together powerfully until you feel your arm muscles contract. Hold the prayer hands pushed together for 20 seconds. Release and repeat the sequence until you feel a little more Zen.

15) Park in the farthest part of the lot.

16) Swivel your chair from side to side. Swish back and forth 15 times.

17) Download an app that turns your screen to black, reminding you to exercise when it does.

18) Try tricep dips, which can be done almost anywhere, even in a cubicle. Using a sturdy desk or a non-rolling chair, sit at the very edge and place hands on each side of your body while gripping the chair's edge. With your feet planted on the floor a step or two away from the desk or chair, straighten up your arms to lift up your body. Next, bend your arms to reach a 90-degree angle so that your body dips down, hold, and re-

straighten while keeping your body raised above the chair. Complete 8-10 reps.

19) Wall sits are great for building strength and endurance. Standing with your back against the wall, bend your knees and slide your back down the wall until your thighs are parallel to the floor. Sit and hold for 30-60 seconds. For extra burn, cross your right ankle over your left knee, hold for 15 seconds, then switch!

20) Work at home? Get a book holder for your stationary bicycle. It works great for iPads, too.

21) Raise both shoulders up toward your ears, hold for 5 seconds, and then relax. Repeat 15 times.

22) Wall Push Ups: Standing one to two feet from a sturdy wall, lean forward until your palms are flush against the wall, with your arms straight and parallel to the ground. Next, bend your elbows to bring your body towards the wall, hold for two seconds, and then push back to the starting position. Complete 12-15 reps.

23) Standing with arms by your sides and palms facing behind, pulse your arms backwards for five seconds. Release and repeat for 12-15 reps. For best results, make sure to keep your arms long and straight!

24) Don't just stand around, like at a printer. Try calf raises. Standing with feet shoulder-width apart, press up onto your tippy toes, pause at the top, and then lower back down. Repeat for three sets of 12-15 reps, or until the printing, faxing or scanning is done.

25) Try this isometric glutes exercise. Simply squeeze your buttocks for 5-10 seconds, and release. Repeat until the meeting wraps up or your glutes get tired.

When you're ready to go the next step

As you become increasingly fit, you may want to up the ante. Two ways to do that in a healthy way are to introduce H.I.I.T. and to add weights.

1. Chase the Rabbit (a.k.a. High Intensity Interval Training, or H.I.I.T.)

Another exercise tip from Dr. John Douillard (www.lifespa.com) is to "Chase the Rabbit," a 12-minute High Intensity Interval Training (H.I.I.T.) technique.

The approach is built upon the science of heart rate variability.

He describes it like this:

"Historically, we would exercise as a way of survival. Hunting a rabbit wouldn't require 45 minutes in your heart rate training zone three times a week. It would require multiple sprints that would last about a minute, followed by periods of rest while you wait for the rabbit to show again.

When we were hunting rabbits, we would sprint and get the heart rate up, then rest and be perfectly still while waiting for it to come out of its hole. Once the rabbit was out, the chase was on again and the heart rate goes up, followed by waiting and resting where the heart rate goes very low."

1) Two-Minute Warm Up. Exercise slowly for two minutes. Be sure to breathe deeply in and out of your nose.

2) Sprint All Out for One Minute. Go all out for a minute, but in a way that you can still breathe deeply in and out through your nose. Be patient with yourself and allow yourself to build up your stamina over time.

3) Recover for One Minute. For one minute, allow your body to recover by going back to the warm up pace. Nasal breathing is still important. Dr. Douillard says, "Nasal Breathing during the recovery will force air into the lower lobes of the lungs allowing for more efficient release of CO_2 and activation of the calming parasympathetic nervous system that predominates in the lower lobes of the lungs. This will help you release toxins and stress."

4) Sprint and Recover three more times. This will bring you to a total of 4 rounds of sprint/recovery. Nasal breathing is still important.

5) Cool Down. You made it! Just repeat Step 1. Exercise slowly with deep nasal breathing for 2 minutes.

"This twelve minute routine can be performed daily or a minimum of 3x/ week for cardiovascular improvements. You can use this as your entire workout or as a cardiovascular warm up before yoga, a bike ride or hiking. In these twelve minutes, you will build your cardiovascular base," according to Douillard.

2. Add Weight Training

Once you've got walking down, add in weight training. Big muscles, little muscles, funny muscles and sleek muscles. Even under the fat, you will be mobilizing those muscles to remember how to burn fat. They will get stronger and more interested in your fat burning concept as you work them. You may not get buns of steel right away, but you will start the fat burning.

Aim for exercises that allow you to do 10 reps (repetitions) without strain. Choose the weight level that allows you to get to 10 reps with a tired but not injured muscle. If you can't lift it more than six times, it is too heavy. If you can lift it 20 times, it is too light. Your body doesn't lie. Listen to it.

My Favorite Walking DVDs

Sometimes, due to weather or time, you just can't get outside. Here are my favorite DVDs for bringing walking inside.

1) Debbie Rocker

- Walking for Weight Loss
- Walk, Sculpt and Tone
- Total Body Challenge: Walk
- Note: Her DVDs come with audio CDs that you can add to your iPhone or iPod for walking outdoors.

2) Leslie Sansone

- Walk at Home

3) Anything from Jillian Michaels

- Generally more overall fitness than walking, but good motivation

The benefits of exercise aren't measured just by a scale, but by a better working body.

5

Step 5
Slash the Sugar

The time has come to
Slash the Sugar.

I know you might not believe it, but if you've followed the Simply Sugar Free steps so far, your body and your brain should be ready for this important step.

First you need to become your own Sugar Sleuth, finding all "sugar" in your diet.

Next you have to decide which approach to eliminating sugar is best for you: Cold Turkey or Easy Does It.

And then you need to slay the Sugar Monster for good!

Let's get started.

What is "sugar" anyway?

You know the Nitty Gritty about sugar. That it consists of two molecules: fructose and glucose. That fructose gives it its sweetness. That glucose provides energy to your cells. And that starches are just long strings of glucose molecules.

Now you need to become your own Sugar Sleuth … sniffing out sugars with the potential to be addictive to you, no matter what they are called.

The words "syrup", "sweetener" and anything ending in "ose" can usually be assumed to be "sugar" and therefore potentially addictive to you.

Sometimes sugar even masquerades under more healthy-sounding names, such as honey, maple syrup, agave nectar and "organic dehydrated cane juice".

Don't be fooled. These are sugar.

Sometimes fruit juice concentrates are used as sweeteners, which sound wholesome. But by the time they are "concentrated" very little remains but the sugar.

If a label says "no added sugars" it should not contain any of the "No Go" sugars in the table, although the food could contain naturally-occurring sugars (such as lactose in milk).

And then there's the whole debate about sugar substitutes. There isn't anything much more controversial than sugar substitutes … natural or not.

Here's my take on the issue: The best end state is to get any sweetness you want from fresh whole foods. Period.

But it may be that the path from totally addicted to Simply Sugar Free passes through stages of sugar substitutes. Just sayin' … (In the world of drug addiction, there is a theory called Harm Reduction. It's about meeting drug users where they are. Using sugar substitutes to help sugar addicts through the process is similar to some of their theories about helping drug addicts through their process.)[19]

For me, I went through stages of alternative sweeteners. I'm happy to say that now, after seven years, I am weaned from them as well. So, while I don't encourage the use of alternative sweeteners, they may serve a purpose in the process of weaning yourself off sugar.

Here is my chart of **Go | No Go | It Depends** "sugars". Note that the chart changes over time as new commercial products are introduced into the marketplace.

Go	No Go		It Depends ...
Barley Malt Syrup	Agave Nectar	Lacitol	Acesulfame
Dextrose*	Coconut Palm	Litesse	potassium (Sunett)
Glucose*	Sugar/Syrup	Maltitol	Alitame
Glucose Syrup*	Corn Syrup	Mannitol	Aspartame (Equal)
Lactose	Dried Cane Juice	Maple Syrup	Aspartame-
Maltose	Fructose	Molasses	acesulfame
Maltodextrin	Fruit Juice Extract	Polydextrose	Cyclamates
Maltodextrose	Golden Syrup	Resistant Dextrin	Date Sugar
Rice Malt Syrup	High Fructose Corn	Sorbitol	Erythritol
	Syrup (HFCS)	Sucrose (Table	Neotame
* Fructose Fanatics	Honey	Sugar)	Saccharin
may be able to	Inulin	Wheat Dextrin	Stevia (Truvia)
tolerate these, but	Isomalt	Whey Low	Sucralose (Splenda)
Glucose Gluttons			Xylitol
may find them			
addictive.			

Cold Turkey or Easy Does It?

Because we are all individual with individual biochemistries, there is no "one" way to Slash the Sugar. Some people prefer to go Cold Turkey. Others prefer an Easy Does it approach.

In the end, you have to do what works for you. Use your workbook to Find Your Frequency. Look at your Unplanned Eating and its causes. You will find clues to help you figure out which strategy will work best for you.

Some people like Going Cold Turkey. Just like that. (My anecdotal observation is that this approach works better for men, than women. I don't know why.)

Personally, Cold Turkey wasn't workable for me. I found that I had to tackle one meal at a time, finding the foods that would work for me, then moving on to the next meal.

Many diets promote an 80/20 or 90/10 approach of eating healthy most of the time, but taking breaks once in awhile. Or having one cheat meal a day or week. Or 5:2, eating well for five days and restricting for two.

For some people this will work.

But if you're a Sugar Addict, you're likely to find that this is the equivalent of wearing a sign that says "Bang head here." You will likely find that it is difficult to break the addictive cycle while consuming the substance. For you, abstaining may actually be much simpler (once you are de-toxed). Remember, the Simply Sugar Free Process is focused on recovery from addiction, not dieting.

I, for one, can not consume sugar in moderation. I have learned that about myself through the Simply Sugar Free Process. I am at my best when all sugar and sugar substitutes are off limits. No negotiating with myself. No slippery slopes for me. My goal is zero added sugar. Zero sugar substitutes. Fresh fruit is my only allowable sugar. (Well, once in awhile I do indulge in teeny tiny amounts of dried fruit such as an add-in to a large green salad.)

It's taken time to get here. But it's where I belong. So although I didn't go Cold Turkey, I have ended up Cold Turkey.

For me, it's just easier this way. For you, it may not be. I need a clear, non-negotiable line over which I do not cross. That way I don't have to spend a lot of time arguing with myself. I know my limits. It is easier for me to abstain, than to spend time figuring out where the boundaries are.

If you drink several sugary beverages each day, or tend to eat mostly processed foods full of added sugars, you may do best gradually decreasing the number of sodas you drink each day, and replace sugary foods with healthy ones. This might ease cravings and make the transition to a healthier lifestyle easier. Or not. You'll know.

There's no right way or wrong way. It's just what works for you. People tend to get dogmatic about the approaches. Just listen to yourself.

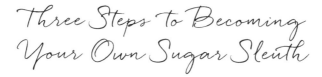

Three Steps To Becoming Your Own Sugar Sleuth

1. Cut Overts; Find and Reduce Coverts

Sometimes sugar hides in plain sight, you know, like cupcakes and candy bars. These are what I call the "Overts" … no one has to tell you there is sugar in most sweet things.

So that's a good place to start. Take the Overts out first, because they are easiest to find.

But then you have to move on to the trickier places that sugar hides … in ketchup, yogurt and even chicken noodle soup!

Finding the "covert" places that sugar hides is more difficult. But if you read labels, know what you're looking for, and don't try to fool yourself … you'll eventually know where to find where sugar is hiding.

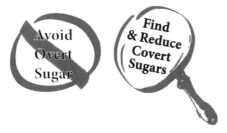

2. No more than 10 grams of sugar per serving

It's best to avoid food with labels at all. But that's not always practical.

So if a food has a label, use the information to your advantage!

Avoid food with more than 10 grams of sugar per serving.

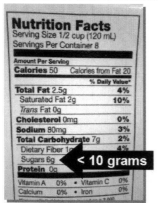

Now, you may have to test your threshold on this one. During the WEAN Phase of the Simply Sugar Free Process you may want to target as close to zero as possible to help you sort out your Red foods.

But during the LEAN phase, you may find that you can add in certain foods. And perhaps under certain conditions. For example, the impact of sugar on an empty stomach is much different than the impact on a full stomach. You may only be able to handle 4 or 5 grams of sugar on an empty stomach, but may be able to handle more as dessert at the end of a meal. When your stomach is full the other foods slow down the blood sugar spike.

Remember, N+1. Keep testing.

3. No sugar listed in the top four ingredients

Ingredients are listed in descending order by weight. If you see sugar (and by that I mean ANY of the "No Go" sugars in the table) listed among the first few ingredients, the product is likely to be high in added sugar.

But beware: manufacturers can (and do) list different sugars separately.

So sometimes even if sugar isn't listed in the top four ingredients, it may appear several different times under different names as shown in the list of ingredients for a breakfast cereal on this slide.

P.S. It's also a good idea to avoid food with more than five ingredients … it's probably highly processed and probably contains one or more types of sugar!

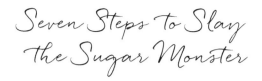

Seven Steps To Slay The Sugar Monster

Now that you know how to seek out and find sugar, here are some ways to hold the Sugar Monster at bay.

1. Don't drink sugar or HFCS.

Ever.

Everyone agrees that one of the biggest contributors to the obesity epidemic is the amount of sugar and HFCS in soda, fruit juices and sports/energy drinks.

Good alternatives are water, green tea and herbal tea. You can also dilute fruit juice half and half with water or seltzer.

P.S. Turning to artificial sweeteners is usually a bad idea. There is much conflicting information about them as well, but many researchers believe that they keep you primed to wanting sweet foods.

2. Eat food that you like.

Because if you don't like what you eat you won't make it part of a permanent lifestyle change!

Keep experimenting and trying new foods. Add ones that you like to the Green Light column in your Red Light | Yellow Light | Green Light Tracker.

Food you like too much should probably be removed from your environment. If you've overeaten it once, you'll probably do it again! Add those to your Red Light column.

3. Trick your taste buds.

Use fresh herbs and spices to trick your taste buds into thinking you're eating something sweet.

Try adding cinnamon, ginger, clove or nutmeg to coffee, cereals or any other dishes or drinks that could use an extra kick.

Add naturally sweet foods to your daily diet to satisfy your sweet tooth and to crowd out less healthy foods.

- Corn, carrots, onions, beets, winter squashes, sweet potatoes and yams are sweet when cooked.

- Turnips, parsnips and rutabagas are slightly less sweet when cooked.
- Some other vegetables don't taste sweet, but have a similar effect on the body in that they maintain blood sugar levels, reduce sweet cravings and break down animal foods in the body. They include red radishes, daikon radish, green cabbage and burdock root.

The good news is that your taste buds will recalibrate over time.

Fruit wasn't sweet enough when I was eating sweets every day. Now it is, because my taste buds have changed. Everyone's do when they change their eating habits, especially when dropping certain foods, like I did with sugar.

When you eat more sugar and fat, that's what will taste best to you. Get rid of the sugar and fat and you won't even like the stuff if you go back.

4. Chew.

Your stomach does not have teeth!

Whole foods must be mixed with saliva and chewed until they become liquid to release their full nutritional value.

In addition, the more that carbohydrates are chewed, the sweeter they become as the starches are broken down into glucose molecules.

To get into the habit of chewing correctly, count the chews in each bite. Aim for 30 to 50 times.

It helps if you put your fork down between bites.

5. Drink more water.

Your brain and body will thank you for it!

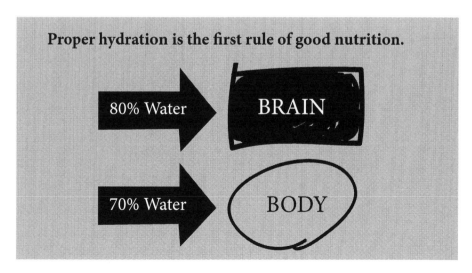

Proper hydration is the first rule of good nutrition.

80% Water → BRAIN

70% Water → BODY

Drink plenty of water, green tea and not too many calories.

One rule of thumb is to drink half your weight in ounces every day.

And remember that not all liquids are created equal! It's best to drink liquids that are free of artificial sweeteners, sugar, much caffeine, and alcohol.

Even slight dehydration increases the body's stress hormones. When this happens, you get irritable and you don't think as well. Over time increased levels of stress hormones are associated with memory problems and obesity.

Dehydration also makes your skin look older and more wrinkled.[20]

6. Get some sunshine.

Sunshine stimulates the production of Vitamin D. And Vitamin D is required for the production of dopamine.

We can get some Vitamin D from food, but most of our Vitamin D is made in the body when our skin is exposed to sunlight. If you spend the daylight hours locked away in an artificially lit office, there's a good chance you don't produce enough Vitamin D.

Try eating your lunch outside in the sun as often as possible, or consider a Vitamin D supplement.

7. Sleep.

There's nothing simpler to keep cravings under control and your leptin levels high (remember, that's your satiety hormone): sleep well.

When you go to sleep, your leptin levels naturally rise. Your body knows to cut down your hunger while you're resting so that hunger won't wake you up. But if you cut your sleeping short, your body tries to adjust by making you hungry again.

Research has found that shorter sleep periods (6 hours or less):
- Lower overall daily leptin levels[21]
- Cause an increase in appetite[22]
- Make you crave carbs and other fattening foods[23]

Reasons to get more sleep:
- Adequate sleep reduces Ghrelin levels and increases the Leptin levels in your blood, which results in a decrease of appetite.
- Getting sufficient sleep reduces hunger and will therefore assist you in losing weight.

6

Step 6:
Love Yourself Silly

Fill the Well with Simple Pleasures

By this point in the Simply Sugar Free Process you should be reaping the rewards of the seeds you have sown.

1) You're eating breakfast every day with at least 20 grams of protein.

2) You've found your frequency, what foods to eat when.

3) You're added more fruits and vegetables into your diet.

4) You're moving at least an hour a day.

5) You're weaning off whites, both sugar and starches.

As a result you are well on your way to balancing your blood sugar and healing your brain chemistry.

But there's one last step, one that is critical to maintaining your momentum and transitioning from the WEAN to LEAN Lifestyle:

Love yourself silly, every day!

Now how's that for an easy-to-swallow prescription for a fun and fulfilled life?

With dopamine and blood sugar now working for you instead of against you, there's one more piece of brain chemistry to optimize: naturally increasing your endorphins (specifically, beta-endorphins) to fortify you against the ups and downs of everyday life.

What are Endorphins?

Endorphins are chemicals used by our bodies as a type of mood and pain regulator. They reduce the feeling of pain, and offset it with a sense of increased happiness, excitement and feeling good, both emotionally and physically.

There are five endorphins, but it's beta-endorphin that helps maintain homeostasis when an outside factor, such as pain, is felt in the body. Beta-endorphin has approximately 80 times the analgesic potency of morphine. (Remember them from breakfast? They're what give you the fake high if you put off eating breakfast.)

Endorphins activate our brain's "reward path." The so called "runner's high" that encourages seasoned runners to get up at six in the morning to jog a couple miles is an example of endorphin release. It is also the chemical that helps a hiker with a broken leg walk for miles until he can get to safety.

Some of us are born with Low Endorphin Levels

Some people are born with low levels of beta-endorphin (notoriously children of alcoholics). If you are one of them:

- You feel anxious and are more aware of pain than people with higher levels of BE.
- You crave fat and fatty foods, such as fries, cheese, creamy sauces, margarine, butter, fried chicken, potato chips and chocolate. Eating these foods causes a release of beta endorphins and you'll feel pleasure. (Exercise, by releasing fat from within the body, raises endorphins and causes the same mood changes.)
- You are depressed, have chronic unexplained pain, and a low tolerance for pain. In many instances, low levels of endorphins are misdiagnosed as depressive disorders.

But the good news is that you can increase your endorphin baseline by introducing gently pleasing activities into your life. How sweet a prescription for happiness is that!

Increasing your beta-endorphin baseline does two important things:

1) The higher baseline makes your life every day more enjoyable. Rather than being depressed and anxious, you will be calm and happy.

2) When something big comes along that used to have the potential to trip your dopamine addiction switch, there will be a much smaller spike in

BE from your new baseline. This makes it less likely that the BE spike will trigger the addictive dopamine release.

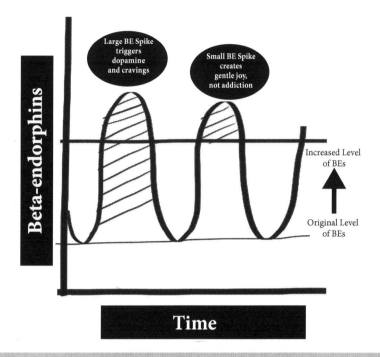

The Good News: Endorphins are not Addictive!

Endorphins affect us like codeine or morphine, but without the addiction.

When endorphins lock into the opioid receptors, they are almost immediately broken down by enzymes, allowing them to be recycled and reused down the road.

However, when similarly shaped but chemically different opiates lock into these same receptors, they are resistant to the enzymes and continue reactivating the receptors over and over, extending the "high" and increasing euphoric feelings, as well as the likelihood of dependence.[24]

365 Ways To Love Yourself Silly

So there's no time like the present to get started loving yourself silly!

Here are 365 ideas to keep you going for a year. Read through the list, or just drop your finger on a page and pick one.

1) Create an at-home spa experience. See the simple and inexpensive / Home Spa Recipes included in the recipe section.

2) Wear silk. There is just something about silk that says "I love you."

3) Enjoy hot water. Every day. Squeezed from a sponge against your belly, down your arms. Hot water pressed against your face. Get lost in water.

4) Try the 4-7-8 Breathing Technique. Watch it demonstrated by Dr. Andrew Weil here: http://www.drweil.com/drw/u/VDR00112/The-4-7-8-Breath-Benefits-and-Demonstration.html. Inhale quietly through your nose to a count of 4. Hold for 7. Exhale through your mouth for 8. Unlike tranquilizing drugs, which are often effective when you first take them but then lose their power over time, this exercise is subtle when you first try it but gains in power with repetition and practice, according to Dr. Weil.

5) Build an altar. Worship you.

6) Find a beautiful cookie jar. Fill it with affirmations instead of cookies ☺

7) Pamper your feet. Rub them. Oil them. Behold them. They have carried you many places.

8) Dance alone, for yourself, in the dark. Move like you do in your dreams. Sweat it out. Get out of breath. Read more about the power of Dancing Your Bliss here: http://www.dancingyourbliss.com/. Go to one of Rachel's workshops. Buy one of her CDs if you can't.

9) Drip rose oil into your palms and place them on your face. Scent is love.

10) Buy expensive jeans and love how you look in them.

11) Take selfies. Share them. Or keep them for yourself. You need no external validation. Keep an entire folder of pictures just of you. For only you.

12) Go skinny dipping.

13) Tell your story. Re-tell your story. Get sick of telling your story. Make up a new story.

14) If you don't have a Pinterest account, create one. Look at pretty pictures of things that please you.

15) Rub coconut oil. All over. Everywhere.

16) Wear black lace.

17) Try Breath Counting. Sit in a comfortable position with your spine straight and head inclined slightly forward. Gently close your eyes and take a few deep breaths. Then let the breath come naturally without trying to influence it. Ideally it will be quiet and slow, but the depth and rhythm may vary.

    • To begin the exercise, count "one" to yourself as you exhale.
    • The next time you exhale, count "two," and so on up to "five."
    • Then begin a new cycle, counting "one" on the next exhalation.
    • Never count higher than "five," and count only when you exhale. Try to do 10 minutes of this form of meditation.

18) Follow Jena La Flamme on-line. Pleasure is her expertise! Sign up for her free newsletter at http://www.pleasurableweightloss.com/.

19) Go for a run in the rain.

20) Get lost in the city or in the forest with a pen and paper. Listen. Write.

21) Kiss yourself in the mirror every single day.

22) Every day write yourself a note that asks "What do you want?" Answer it in your journal.

23) Sign up for a workshop at the Omega Institute http://www.eomega.org/. Let someone else cook for you and take care of you for a few days while you learn something new. On the East Coast you can get there by Amtrak … let someone else do the driving, too!

24) Write poetry on your body. In black ink. Let it wear away on its own. In its own time. In its own space. Until it does. Let your body drink in the words.

25) Get tarot cards. Read them daily.

26) Feel your hands. Hold your hands in your hands. Interlace your fingers together. Smell your hands. Rub your palms together. Get them hot. Place on them your cheeks. Press your fingers together and then press them against your lips. Kiss your hands. Run your fingers through your hair.

27) Buy some really pretty rings and get married along the waterside to your one and only you.

28) Take a nap.

29) Get a massage.

30) Read easy, fun reads for a change, not self-help or professional books!

31) Snuggle with the cat (or dog or baby or kids).

32) Give or get hugs.

33) Take a long walk and/or hike.

34) Take a bubble bath.

Get Better at What You're Good At to Bring Joy

It's important to discover your strengths because the luckiest people are the ones who get to say to themselves every day: "Today, I had the opportunity to do what I am most invigorated by and what I do best."

If you look at the happiest and most successful women—whether they are working or not, or have families or don't—they seem to realize that the challenge of life is not to juggle; the challenge is to catch—to select a few clear, strong moments from each aspect of your life and reach for those, draw them in to you. If you want to live a life that fulfills you, then you need to know, in each part of your life, which are the specific moments that really renew your energy and bring you joy, and go after them. You want to imbalance your life toward creating more of those specific moments. It's a very different approach from what most people are taught, according to Marcus Buckingham, author of Find Your Strongest Life: What the Happiest and Most Successful Women Do Differently.

What are the SIGNs of your strengths?

There's a simple acronym to help you recognize the signs of strength: SIGN.

S— Success: Do you feel a sense of accomplishment about finishing this task?

I— Instinct: Do you instinctively look forward to this task?

G— Growth: Are your synapses firing? Are you mentally focused?

N— Needs: Does this task fulfill one of your needs?

People feel the need to be well-rounded because society gives us that message from the time we're schoolchildren. If a child comes home with a report card that shows five A's and only one C, chances are the parents are going to spend the majority of their time talking about improving on the C, rather than on celebrating the A's. This continues into our working lives, where performance reviews often consist of a brief pat on the back for those areas that are working well and then a substantial focus on our "areas of opportunity."

We internalize this. The problem with focusing on what doesn't work is that attention amplifies everything. If you focus on the problem with the intent of fixing it, despite your best intentions, that problem becomes magnified. Instead, we need to shift our focus and ask, "What's working well, and how can I get more of that?"

Marcus Buckingham is a leadership expert, internationally renowned speaker and New York Times bestselling author of several books, including First, Break All the Rules; Now Discover Your Strengths and Find Your Strongest Life: What the Happiest and Most Successful Women Do Differently.

P.S. When I took Buckingham's "Strengths Accelerator" I came out as a Creator and Stimulator. Guess I was meant to write and coach ☺

35) Watch movies. Happy movies.

36) Order dinner in.

37) Just say no.

38) Buy yourself flowers.

39) Try Alternate Nostril Breathing.

- Sit in a comfortable position. Inhale.
- Gently close off your left nostril with your right pinky.
- Exhale a long gentle exhale through your right nostril.
- Then inhale up the right nostril with a long inhale. At the top, momentarily close off both nostrils with your right thumb and pinky.
- Open the left nostril and exhale. Then inhale up the left nostril, close off both nostrils and open and exhale down the right.
- Keep moving your breath in this pattern down one side and then up and switch.
- Continue for 5 minutes.

- A picture is worth a thousand words. Here's a video that demonstrates this type of breathing: http://www.amazon.com/Dr-John-Douillard-Ayurveda-Stress/dp/B000YV1KYU

40) Sip a mug of hot, soothing tea.

41) Play in the snow.

42) Dig your toes into the sand.

43) Feel the sun (or rain) on your face.

44) Hold hands.

45) Meditate.

46) Get a facial.

47) Listen to your favorite music.

48) Watch something inspirational on http://www.ted.com/talks/browse.

49) Make a Delights List. Do something on your Delights list.

50) Learn more about meditation at The Chopra Center http://www.chopra.com/. Several times a year they do free 21-day on-line meditation series. Or buy a CD to keep at home.

51) Get Acupuncture.

52) Journal.

53) Turn off the computer, cell phone and TV for 24 hours.

54) Go on a retreat.

55) Sit and people watch.

56) Garden.

57) Do something creative (draw, knit, cross-stitch, paint, cook, write, color, make a collage, etc.).

58) Daydream.

59) Dance with a child.

60) Have a Harry Potter movie marathon.

61) Take a mental health day from work.

62) Keep your daily to-do list to 3 items or less.

63) Swing on the swings.

64) Have energy work done.

65) Do an at-home cleanse with Dr. John Douillard. I do his five-day Short Home Cleanse twice a year. Get the .pdf here: http://lifespa.com/cleansing/short-home-cleanse/

66) Have a laugh fest with your best friend.

67) Eat simply.

68) Break up with your TV.

69) Allow yourself to cry and experience your emotions.

70) Join a support group.

71) Get a pedicure (or manicure).

72) Tell yourself "I love you".

73) Browse your favorite bookstore (or music store).

74) Have a game night with friends.

75) Write thank you notes to those who have touched your life and inspired you.

76) Spend the day exploring your town – go places you don't normally go.

77) Practice random acts of kindness & senseless acts of beauty.

78) Write a love letter to someone you love.

79) Write a love letter to yourself.

80) Have a "Freedom from Self-Improvement Day".

81) Color (try going outside the lines – its fun!).

82) Keep a gratitude journal.

83) Take a walk and take pictures of all you see that delights you.

84) Find and notice something beautiful every day.

85) Do something badly. Keep doing it.

86) Admire beautiful artwork.

87) Do absolutely nothing.

88) Do one brave thing everyday.

89) Play.

90) Treat yourself to something.

91) Wear something that makes you feel beautiful or handsome and confident.

92) Stay in your PJs all day.

93) Say I love you every day.

94) Jump in piles of leaves.

95) Quit the job you hate that drains you.

96) Say YES to what you truly love.

97) Give yourself permission.

98) Let go of belongings you no longer love or use (even family heirlooms). Also applies to relationships.

99) Hire someone to clean your house.

100) Hire someone to mow your lawn.

101) Let go of your story.

102) Laugh.

103) Be generous.

104) Lie in the grass and watch the clouds.

105) Take a long walk with your dog.

106) Ride a horse.

107) Give up New Year's Resolutions.

108) Stop drinking caffeine.

109) Dance around your house.

110) Forgive others.

111) Forgive yourself.

112) Make a list of the things you want to do in your lifetime. . Do one of those things. And then do another.

113) Eat healthy, whole foods.

114) Eat something unhealthy (but sugar free!) AND enjoy it without self-criticism or guilt.

115) Watch cartoons.

116) Read the comics.

117) Smile for no reason.

118) Call the friends you've been meaning to call.

119) Go complaint free.

120) Schedule a day of no schedule.

121) Go boat riding.

122) Buy yourself a cheery balloon.

123) Walk naked around the house.

124) Give generously of yourself and your resources.

125) View everything and everyone you meet with gratitude.

126) Live today happily without focusing on your problems.

127) Hum or sing a happy song.

128) Foster a sense of humor.

129) Smell some flowers.

130) Call your family and tell them how much you appreciate them.

131) Treat yourself to regular daily quiet time - study, pray, meditate; recharge yourself.

132) Experiment with new ways to exercise. Try yoga, Pilates, martial arts, walking, running, bicycling, rollerblading, swimming, dancing, weight lifting or competitive sports.

133) Scrub your entire body with a hot, damp washcloth in the morning and/or evening to increase your circulation.

134) Avoid wearing synthetic or woolen clothing directly on the skin. As much as possible, wear 100% cotton clothing, especially for undergarments.

135) Avoid excessive jewelry on your fingers, wrists and neck; fewer rings, bracelets, necklaces, earrings and piercings. This allows your natural energy to flow more freely.

136) Avoid chemically perfumed cosmetics.

137) Use natural toothpastes.

138) Keep your home in good order, including kitchen, bathroom, bedroom, and living rooms. You are your home.

139) If possible, include large green plants in every room of your home and office to freshen and enrich the oxygen content of the air.

140) Minimize television watching, or at least keep a good distance away from the television.

141) Avoid cooking with electricity, especially microwave ovens. Convert to gas when practical.

142) Avoid water with chlorine and fluoride. Use spring water or a good-quality water filter.

143) Chew your food well, 30 seconds per mouthful or more, until it becomes liquid.

144) Offer thanks before and after meals.

145) Do your best to be on good terms with people, especially your boyfriend or girlfriend, husband or wife, parents, children, brothers, sisters, friends, and co-workers. Communicate with them regularly in person, via telephone or via email.

146) Create a positive attitude and wonderful environment around you, and enjoy the process of becoming healthier and happier every step of the way!

147) Oil up your body and give yourself a massage.

148) View each person in your life as a gift to teach you lessons. Ask yourself: why is this person in my life?

149) Practice the four agreements from Don Miquel Ruiz: be impeccable with your word, don't take anything personally, don't make assumptions, and always do your best.

150) Purge your closet regularly. Make room for more. Stop hanging onto the past.

151) Light candles often (soy if possible).

152) Take a bath instead of a shower.

153) Make your bed.

154) Rid your home of chemical-type cleaners and opt for natural, enzymatic or organic options.

155) Drink alkaline water when possible.

156) Perform a random act of kindness on a daily basis.

157) Tip more, even if they don't deserve it.

158) Walk in the mountains.

159) Go play outside.

160) Read: the paper, a novel, something new.

161) Practice speaking nicely to yourself.

162) Write or journal.

163) Draw a picture.

164) Paint.

165) Buy yourself something nice.

166) Lie on your back outside and stare at the clouds.

167) Learn a new song, in Français.

168) Play in the rain.

169) Cry. Really, cry.

170) Smile at and compliment a complete stranger.

171) Ride your bike.

172) Send love to someone.

173) Give to someone randomly without them knowing, and don't ever tell them.

174) Pray.

175) Go rock climbing.

176) Cook a great meal with great friends.

177) Snorkel in the ocean.

178) Climb a tree.

179) Sit outside and watch some birds.

180) Walk outside barefoot.

181) Dance like no one is watching you.

182) Visit a garden.

183) Each time you wear something, put it back in your closet on the hanger backwards. At the end of the season, you can tell what you've worn and what you haven't. Consider getting rid of what you haven't worn.

184) Visit an art gallery.

185) Learn something brand new.

186) Go skiing or snowboarding.

187) Play in the sand.

188) Drink some water.

189) Lie on the couch and look outside.

190) Sit with yourself for 20 minutes with no noise or distractions.

191) Swim naked.

192) Praise yourself.

193) Connect deeply with another.

194) Leave a thank you note for awesome service.

195) Play some golf.

196) Read "The Monk Who Sold His Ferrari" by Robin Sharma.

197) Read "The War of Art".

198) Help someone without expecting anything in return.

199) Cook something delightful.

200) Brush your hair for a few minutes (or massage your head).

201) Breathe deeply.

202) Listen to some calming music.

203) Spend time with some animals.

204) Donate some books or clothes to a shelter, hospital, nursing home, etc.

205) Switch your fried eggs for poached or hard-boiled.

206) Let go of negative self-talk. Bashing yourself on a daily basis takes a toll. When you hear negative self-talk, say "cancel cancel" followed by a positive comment to condition yourself to speak positively.

207) Eat extra greens.

208) Stretch your muscles.

209) Collect evidence of love and bring back proof through pictures, clippings or words to create a reminder board.

210) Laugh so hard you cry.

211) Go see a movie.

212) Create a vision board using old magazines.

213) Go on a picnic.

214) Thank the earth and plant a tree.

215) Visit your farmers market.

216) Forgive. Yourself and everyone else.

217) Listen to your favorite music.

218) Make a list of ten things you're good at or that you like about yourself when you're feeling good, and keep it with you to read when you're feeling upset.

219) Enjoy a long, warm bubble bath.

220) Relax outside.

221) Practice feeling contented.

222) Do a physical activity of your choice.

223) Say a spiritual prayer of your choice.

224) Practice diaphragmatic breathing. Google for instructions.

225) Do stretching exercises.

226) Reflect on your positive qualities: "I am…".

227) Watch the sunrise or set.

228) Concentrate on a relaxing scene.

229) Create a collage representing "the real you".

230) Reflect on: "I appreciate ..."

231) Attend a favorite athletic event.

232) Do something adventurous!

233) Read a special magazine.

234) Play a musical instrument.

235) Do a spiritual meditation.

236) Learn a new skill.

237) See a special play, movie or concert.

238) Work out with weights.

239) Ride a bike or motorcycle.

240) Make a nutritious meal.

241) Swim, float, wade, relax in a pool, or on the beach.

242) Do aerobics/dance.

243) Visit a special place you enjoy.

244) Smile and say "I love myself."

245) Take time to smell the roses.

246) Imagine yourself achieving your goals and dreams.

247) Reflect on your most enjoyable memories.

248) Practice yoga.

249) Relax in a whirlpool /sauna.

250) Enjoy a cool, refreshing glass of water or juice.

251) Enjoy the beauty of nature.

252) Count your blessings: "I am thankful for …"

253) Play as you did as a child.

254) Star gaze.

255) Stay up late or get up early!

256) Window shop.

257) Daydream.

258) Tell yourself the loving words you want to hear from others.

259) Attend a special workshop.

260) Go sailing/paddle boating.

261) Reward yourself with a special gift you can afford.

262) Take yourself on a vacation.

263) Create with clay/pottery.

264) Practice positive affirmations.

265) Pet an animal.

266) Watch your favorite TV show.

267) Reflect on your successes: "I CAN…."

268) Make a bouquet of flowers.

269) Make yourself something nice.

270) Visit a park/woods/forest.

271) Read positive, motivational literature.

272) Reflect on: "What I value most in life…"

273) Go on a picnic in a beautiful setting.

274) Enjoy a gourmet cup of herbal tea or coffee.

275) Practice a relaxation exercise.

276) Practice the art of forgiveness.

277) Treat yourself to a nutritious meal at a favorite restaurant.

278) Practice feeling awe for life.

279) Discover a new place.

280) Hug a tree!

281) "Meow" with a cat; "bark "with a dog, "chirp" with a bird !

282) Go out and visit a friend.

283) Invite a friend to visit you at your home.

284) Text message your friends.

285) Spend time with your family.

286) Organize a party.

287) Do something exciting, like surfing, rock climbing, skiing, skydiving, or kayaking, or learn how to do one of these sports.

288) Go to your local playground and join a game being played or watch a game.

289) Go play something you can do by yourself if no one else is around, like basketball, bowling, handball, miniature golf, billiards, or hitting a tennis ball against the wall.

290) Get out of your house, even if you just sit outside in the fresh air.

291) Go for a drive in your car or take a ride on public transportation.

292) Plan a trip to a place you've never been before.

293) Cook your favorite dish or meal.

294) Cook a recipe that you've never tried before.

295) Take a cooking class.

296) Borrow a friend's dog and take it to the park.

297) The average person has an estimated 70,000 thoughts per day. Positive thoughts boost your mood and spirit, and tend to generate even more positivity and happiness in your life. Choose to switch to a happier perception and reach for better thoughts. It takes a little practice, but soon enough, your mind will gravitate to the brighter side of life.

298) Give your pet a bath.

299) Listen to the radio.

300) Play a game with a friend.

301) Play solitaire.

302) Play video games.

303) Go online to chat.

304) Write a letter to someone who has made your life better and tell the person why. (You don't have to send the letter if you don't want to.)

305) Visit your favorite websites.

306) Visit crazy websites and start keeping a list of them.

307) Create your own website.

308) Think of someone who has done something important for you who you've never properly thanked. In a letter, write down exactly what they did and the specific effect it had on your life. Be specific. Write and rewrite it multiple times. Make it powerful and concise. Handwrite the letter or use calligraphy – be creative. Meet with the person face to face, and read them the letter.

309) Create your own online blog.

310) Join an Internet dating service.

311) Sell something you don't want on the Internet.

312) Buy something on the Internet.

313) Do a puzzle with a lot of pieces.

314) Start collecting funny movies to watch when you're feeling overwhelmed with pain.

315) Go shopping.

316) Get a haircut.

317) Go to a library.

318) Go to a bookstore and read.

319) Go to the mall or the park and watch other people; try to imagine what they're thinking.

320) Go to your church, synagogue, temple or other place of worship.

321) Join a group at your place of worship.

322) Write a letter to God, the Universe or whatever Higher Power you believe in.

323) Learn a new language.

324) Write a song.

325) Listen to some upbeat, happy music. Start collecting happy songs for times when you're feeling overwhelmed.

326) Memorize lines from your favorite movie, play or song.

327) Make a movie or video with your phone.

328) Join a public speaking group and write a speech.

329) Participate in a local theater group.

330) Let go of comparing yourself to others. While it's easy to want what others have, comparing yourself is like discarding everything you've got going for you at this very moment.

331) Sing in a local choir.

332) Join a club.

333) Knit, crochet, or sew—or learn how to.

334) Make a scrapbook with pictures.

335) Push your own Pause button. Literally put your index finger to the middle of your forehead and force yourself to pause. (Thanks to Gabrielle Bernstein for this tip. Follow her anywhere online for lots of great ideas! https://www.facebook.com/gabriellebernstein)

336) Paint your nails.

337) Change your hair color.

338) Work on your car, truck, motorcycle or bicycle.

339) Sign up for a class that excites you at a local college, adult school or online.

340) Read a trashy celebrity magazine.

341) Write a letter to a friend or family member.

342) Write a list of the things you like about yourself.

343) Write a poem, story, movie or play about your life or someone else's.

344) Write in your journal or diary about what happened to you today.

345) Write a loving letter to yourself when you're feeling good, and keep it with you to read when you're feeling upset.

346) Paint a picture with your fingers.

347) Share intimate experiences with someone you care about.

348) Make a list of the people you admire and want to be like—they can be real or fictional people throughout history. Describe what you admire about them.

349) Write a story about the craziest, funniest or sexiest thing that ever happened to you.

350) Make a list of 10 things you would like to do before you die.

351) Make a list of 10 celebrities you would like to be friends with and describe why.

352) Massage your face with olive oil for one minute at night after cleansing, remove excess oil with cotton.

353) Create your own list of pleasurable activities.

354) Before you go to bed, write down three good things that happened during the day. Then, write down why each of them happened. Think about the impact these positive events had on your day. How would your day have gone if they didn't happen? Identify three strategies for continuing to live in a state of thankfulness, manifesting more positivity and improvement.

355) Write down each time something good happens, or actions you take to make a bad situation good.

356) What are some of your signature strengths? Brainstorm ways you can use them even more, writing down specific actions you can take. Commit to using your strengths in new ways this week. Carry a small notebook with you and write down each time you complete an action that utilizes your signature strengths.

357) Let go of limiting beliefs. Replace beliefs that just aren't serving you any more and rework them to into self-supporting goals.

358) If you want different results, do something different. But make small changes. There's no need to create chaos in the name of change.

359) Let go of the need to always be right. Would you rather be right or would you rather be happy?

360) When you think you don't have it all, focus on what you have today. Keep a gratitude journal and each day write down five thoughts you are grateful for.

361) Walk with energy and purpose. Make a conscious effort to strut! Even when you're feeling down and discouraged, stand tall and smile! Posture affects your mood; make it work in your favor.

362) Surround yourself with like-minded, uplifting people. People who are vibrating on the same positive frequency will keep you grounded, inspired, and connected to your greater life's purpose. They will help you believe in yourself, too.

363) Do good for someone else. Focus your energy on lifting up someone else and notice how your spirits elevate as well.

364) Experiment with new types of meditation. Search on-line. A good source is www.chopra.com.

365) Experiment with meditating at other times, such as at your desk before a long meeting, after a workout, at bedtime – really, whenever it is safe to close your eyes and allow your concentration to move inward.

7

Resources

Books To Read

- The Bliss Cleanse
    - Lindsey Smith and Lorraine Miller

- The Blood Sugar Solution
    - Mark Hyman

- Body, Mind and Sport
    - John Douillard

- The End of Overeating: Taking Control of the Insatiable American Appetite
    - David Kessler

- Fat Chance: Beating The Odds Against Sugar, Processed Food, Obesity, and Disease
    - Robert Lustig

- Food Rules: An Eater's Manual
    - Michael Pollen

- The Gratitude Journal
    - Lorraine Miller

- The Hunger Fix
    - Pamela Peake

- Integrative Nutrition
    - Joshua Rosenthal

- Junk Foods and Junk Moods
    - Lindsey Smith

- May Cause Miracles
    - Gabrielle Bernstein

- Potatoes not Prozac
  - Kathleen DesMaisons

- Salt Sugar Fat: How the Food Giants Hooked Us
  - Michael Moss

- Spontaneous Happiness
  - Andrew Weil

- Sugar Addicts Total Recovery Program
  - Kathleen DesMaisons

- Sweet Poison: Why Sugar is Making Us Fat
  - David Gillespie

- Why We Get Fat
  - Gary Taubes

People to Follow

David Gillespie

- http://sweetpoison.com.au/

John Douillard

- www.lifespa.com

Kathleen DesMaisons

- www.radiantrecovery.com
- https://twitter.com/radiantrecovery

Mark Hyman

- http://drhyman.com/

Nicole Avena

- http://www.drnicoleavena.com
- https://twitter.com/DrNicoleAvena
- https://www.facebook.com/DrNicoleAvena

Robert Lustig

- https://www.facebook.com/DrRobertLustig

Videos To Watch

The Skinny on Obesity (Six-Part Series)

http://www.youtube.com/watch?v=h0zD1gj0pXk&list=PL89BD934934
EC2AAE&index=7

Sugar: The Bitter Truth (1 hour)

http://www.youtube.com/watch?v=dBnniua6-oM

8

Recipes

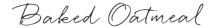

Baked Oatmeal

Ingredients

1 cup rolled oats
1 cup oat bran
1 ½ t baking powder
1 t baking soda
Dash salt
Blend:
2 eggs
½ cup plain yogurt
1 cup milk
½ cup unsweetened applesauce
1 t cinnamon
1 t pumpkin pie spice
½ t nutmeg
1 ½ t sugar-free vanilla flavoring

Method

1) Preheat oven to 350°F.
2) Spray 8" x 8" glass pan with non-stick spray or line with foil.
3) In a bowl, mix together oats, oat bran, baking powder, baking soda, and salt. In another bowl, whisk together eggs, yogurt, milk, applesauce, cinnamon, pumpkin pie spice, nutmeg, and vanilla.
4) Add wet ingredients to dry, stir, and put into pan and into oven immediately.
5) Bake for 25 – 30 minutes, or until top is golden brown and the oatmeal feels firm to the touch.
6) Cool for a few minutes and then turn out of the pan onto a cooling rack.

Serve warm or cold.
Makes 4 – 8 servings.

This recipe can be modified by changing the seasonings, adding berries or nuts, etc. You can also add protein powder to this. If you would like nice, concise, easily-freezable servings, bake in muffin tins for a shorter length of time.

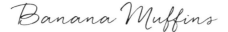

Banana Muffins

Ingredients

1 cup oat flour
1 cup brown rice flour
1 tsp baking soda
1 t salt
2 eggs
3 ripe bananas
1 jar banana baby food
1/2 cup walnut pieces

Method

1) Preheat oven to 350.

2) Mix dry ingredients together in a bowl.

3) In a larger bowl, beat eggs, and mix in bananas one at a time with electric mixer. Then add baby food and mix well.

4) Mix in dry ingredients, a bit at a time, until blended well. Stir in walnut pieces.

5) You can either pour it into an oiled loaf pan and bake for about 50 minutes, or put in an oiled muffin tin and bake for about 20 minutes.

Banana Nut Bread

Ingredients

I 2/3 cups white whole wheat flour or whole wheat pastry flour (or 1 cup oat flour and 2/3 cup brown rice flour)

½ cup butter, softened

2 eggs

2 cups pureed banana

1/3 cup of water

1 ½ scoops of protein powder

2 t orange flavoring

1 t baking soda

½ t salt

¼ t baking powder

½ cup chopped nuts

Method

1) Preheat oven to 350°F.

2) Mix all ingredients together.

3) Pour into non-stick or greased loaf pan and bake for an hour, or until toothpick inserted comes out clean.

Batman Super Hero Super Food Bars

This is from my friend Annie Wagoner on her site Core Nourishment: http://www.yourcorenourishment.com/.

"As a working mom of two, a holistic health counselor, and someone who is passionate about nourishing my kids, I feel like I'm constantly searching for creative and "magical" recipes to fuel my children. With the recent superhero drama in my house, I decided to play with the idea of making Superhero Super-Food Bars for kids. Why not create a whole food bar that literally includes "superfoods" and embodies characteristics of a superhero? Superheroes represent incredible strength (the Hulk), extra stamina (Spiderman), rapid healing powers (Wolverine), flight (Superman), super speed (the Flash)...the list goes on...

So, on a recent rainy afternoon, while Sadie was napping, Jack pulled his chair up to the kitchen counter, grabbed his mixing spoon, and helped me stir up a delicious, whole food Batman bar. What is a Batman bar? Check out our simple recipe:

Ingredients
1 ripe mashed banana
1.5 cup oats
1/4 cup ground flaxseeds
1/4 cup chia seeds
1/2 cup unsweetened shredded coconut
2 scoops hemp protein
1/2 cup raisins (or other dried fruit)
1/2 cup peanut butter (or a nut butter of your choice)
1/2 cup Enjoy Life dairy-free chocolate chips
(or raw cacao nibs if you're sugar sensitive)
1/3 cup maple syrup (optional if you're sugar sensitive)
1/2 t cinnamon
1 t vanilla extract

(These are all estimated amounts since, with Jack, I tend to be a little more lenient about exact measurements :) It makes the experience more authentic and fun. Plus, you can't really go wrong with banana, peanut butter, coconut, and chocolate in the mix :))

197

Method

We threw the dry ingredients in a bowl and then added the wet ingredients, stirred and stirred, taste tested, transferred into an 8x8 baking dish, covered and put in the freezer for an hour or two. The Batman superfood mixture hardened in the freezer enough so that I could cut it into little bars, wrap them individually, and then save them for those emergency moments when we need an extra boost of strength or stamina, or when we want to fly :).

Breakfast Muffins

Method

1) In large bowl combine:
   1-1/2 cups whole wheat flour (or 1 cup brown rice flour and
   1/2 cup of quinoa)
   3/4 cup uncooked oatmeal
   2 t baking powder
   1/2 t salt
   1/2 t baking soda

2) In a glass measuring cup (or small bowl) mix:
   1/2 cup milk (any kind)
   1/4 cup canola oil
   2 eggs

3) Beat these all together. Then pour into dry mixture and blend until moistened.

4) In another medium bowl:
   8 oz. cream cheese (regular or Neufchatel)
   1-1/2 bananas chopped
   1 t vanilla (or other) flavoring

5) Add to muffin batter but don't blend completely, so there are little bites of mostly cream cheese in the muffins. Spoon into muffin cups. Bake at 350 degrees Fahrenheit for 20 minutes.

Makes one dozen.

Flavor Variations:

- Add 1 cup shredded cheddar cheese and 6 pieces fried, crumbled bacon to the dry mixture before adding liquids.
- Add chopped strawberries or other berries to cream cheese mixture before adding to the batter, can also add unsweetened coconut.
- Add a heaping spoonful of peanut or almond butter to the cream cheese mixture.
- Cover the tops of each muffin with pecan halves or unsweetened coconut before baking.

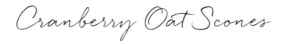

Cranberry Oat Scones

Ingredients

1 ¾ cups whole wheat pastry flour
3 shakes salt
¾ t baking soda
1 t baking powder
½ cup (1 stick) unsalted butter, cold and cut into small pieces
¾ cup old-fashioned rolled oats
½ cup cranberries, cut in half
Zest of one orange, chopped
OJ and buttermilk to make 2/3 cup (I usually just puree the orange I used for the zest)

Egg Wash:
1 large egg
1 T milk

Method

1) Preheat the oven to 375°F and place rack in center of oven. Line a baking sheet with parchment paper and set aside.

2) In the food processor combine butter, flour, salt, baking soda, and baking powder. Remove and put in mixing bowl and add the rolled oats, cranberries and zest. Mix until combined. Stir in the OJ/butter milk (adding more buttermilk if necessary) and mix just until the dough comes together.

3) Transfer to a lightly floured surface and knead the dough four or five times and then pat, or roll, the dough into a circle that is 7" round and about 1 ½" thick. Cut this circle into 6 triangular sections. Place the scones on the baking sheet. Make an egg wash of one beaten egg mixed with 1 tablespoon milk and brush the tops of the scones with this mixture.

4) Bake for about 15 – 18 minutes or until lightly browned and a tooth pick inserted in the middle comes out clean. Transfer to a wire rack to cool.

Makes 6 scones.

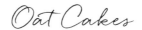

Oat Cakes

Ingredients

10 extra large eggs
16 oz almond milk
1/2 cup slivered almonds
3 scoops protein powder
6 T ground flax seed
3-4.5 cups of dry oats (depending on Old-Fashioned GF Bob's or store brand quick oats, and also on how you want your cakes...lighter or heavier)
3-4 T cinnamon
1 small apple diced really small

Method

Mix all ingredients and let stand for a bit to soften oats, especially if using Bob's OF. You're looking for a soft but not too liquid batter (and you can add oats or milk to fix it).

Use a scant ¼ cup measure to pour them on to a Teflon griddle, four at a time. Flip them over like regular pancakes when they look dry around the edges and bubbly in the middle.

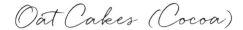

Oat Cakes (Cocoa)

Ingredients

3 cups oats

3 cups sweet potato (cooked)

2 eggs

1 cup natural unsweetened Peanut Butter

1 cup Chocolate Flavored Whey unsweetened Protein Powder

1/2 c plain almond milk

Method

1) Blend potatoes w almond milk and egg so that you can pour them into a bowl with the oats and the peanut butter.

2) Add the protein powder slowly s that it doesn't get lumpy.

3) Bake in a 9 x 13 pan for 40 mins at 350 (until the edges are brown).

- Some people don't add peanut butter and use cooked black beans instead.
- Some people add coconut or coconut milk.
- Some people add oil instead of almond milk.
- Cut up and freeze for protein/healthy carb snacks.

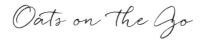

Ingredients

1/3 cup oats
2 egg whites
1/2 scoop of protein powder
Dash of cinnamon
Stevia packet
1/8 t baking powder
Raisins (optional)

Method

1) Mix all ingredients together.
2) Bake at 350 for 15 minutes.

Wrap in foil and store in a plastic baggie.
Double recipe for multiple servings.

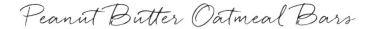

Peanut Butter Oatmeal Bars

Ingredients

½ cup unsweetened applesauce
2 cups of rolled oats
½ cup of sugar-free granola
1 t vanilla flavoring (sugar free)
2 eggs (or ½ cup Eggbeaters)
1 scoop of protein powder
½ cup of unsalted crunchy organic peanut butter

Method

1) Preheat oven to 350°F.

2) Spray an 8" x 8" pan with cooking spray. Spread the mixture out evenly in the pan. Bake for 20 minutes. Remove from oven and let cool. Cut into granola bars.

Makes 8 – 10 bars.
Note: This recipe can be doubled, using a 9" x 13" pan.

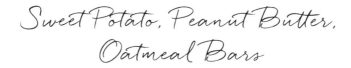

Sweet Potato, Peanut Butter, Oatmeal Bars

Ingredients

    3 cups cooked sweet potato, skin removed
    3 cups quick-cooking rolled oats (raw)
    3/4 cup peanut butter
    1 cup protein powder
    1/2 cup water

Method

1) Preheat oven to 350F.

2) Mash the sweet potatoes in a large mixing bowl with the water, then add the other ingredients and use the masher to blend well. The mixture should be thick but almost pourable.

3) Turn into a greased 9 X13 baking dish, bake at 350F for 45 minutes.

Cool. Cut into 32 squares.
Refrigerate or freeze until ready to use.

Options:

- Try almond butter.
- Play with the proportion of water and the cooking time to make them drier or more moist. Add spices!
- Use pureed black beans in place of some of the sweet potato and oats.

Breakfast Roll-Ups

Method

1) Start with a flatbread or tortilla and spread a little cream cheese on it. Then scramble 3 eggs with a little chopped onion, shredded cheddar, salt and pepper and a little water (makes eggs fluffy) in a non-stick skillet in a little olive oil.

2) Put the eggs on the flatbread or tortilla. You can add a little smoked salmon to it.

3) Roll it up, put it in the microwave and warm for a few seconds to soften the flat bread.

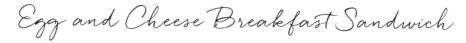

Egg and Cheese Breakfast Sandwich

Ingredients

2 eggs
Shredded cheddar cheese
Light or regular cream cheese
2 slices whole grain bread
Butter for grilling

Method

1) Scramble the eggs with the cheddar cheese, and set them aside.
2) Butter one side of a slice of bread & spread cream cheese on the other side.
3) Put the bread on the frying pan, cream cheese up.
4) Put the scrambled eggs and cheese on top.
5) Butter one side of the remaining slice of bread & spread cream cheese on the other side.
6) Put that slice on top of the eggs, cream cheese down.
7) Grill the sandwich until lightly browned on both sides over medium low heat.

Egg, Cheese and Canadian Bacon Breakfast Sandwich

Method

- Toast a whole-wheat English muffin.
- Melt some cheese on each half.
- Fry an egg with a little bit of olive oil on low heat until the yolk is not runny.
- Add 2 or 3 slices of Canadian bacon (regular or soy-based if you wish).

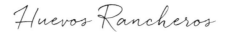

Huevos Rancheros

Ingredients

4 eggs
4 tortillas
1/2 cup cooked black beans
1/2 cup medium salsa

Possible Toppings

Grated cheddar cheese
Chopped scallions
Chopped parsley or cilantro
Tofu or almond milk cheese

Method

1) Heat tortillas in oven or toaster just until soft.
2) Warm salsa and black beans in a nonstick pan.
3) Move to one side. Crack eggs and cook 3-5 minutes to desired firmness.
4) Place two warm tortillas side-by-side on a warmed plate and slide eggs and half the salsa and beans onto the tortillas.
5) Repeat with remaining eggs.
6) Garnish with your choice of toppings.

Banana Walnut Protein-Fortified Oatmeal

Ingredients

1/2 cup raw oats
3 T protein powder (more or less)
1/2 banana
1/4 cup of walnuts
1 cup milk

Method

1) Put all ingredients in a food processor or blender to form a paste.

2) Put the paste In a bowl and mix with 1 cup milk.

3) Cook in the microwave at 50% power for 6 minutes. Stir in some cinnamon and continue cooking for another 3-4 minutes, depending on how you like the texture of your oatmeal.

4) Add milk as desired.

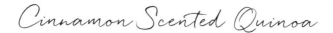

Cinnamon Scented Quinoa

Ingredients

 1 cup quinoa (all red or a mix of red, white, or black)
 1 1/2 cups water
 2 cinnamon sticks
 1/4 t salt

Accompaniments

Broken or chopped walnuts, milk, and flaky sea salt

Method

 1) Wash quinoa and drain.
 2) Combine all ingredients in a heavy medium saucepan and bring to a boil, covered.
 3) Reduce heat to low and cook, covered, until water is absorbed and quinoa is tender, about 20 minutes.
 4) Remove pan from heat and let stand, covered, 5 minutes. Fluff with a fork and keep covered to keep warm. Remove cinnamon sticks.
 5) Divide quinoa among bowls and top with walnuts, milk, and sea salt.

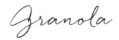

Granola

Ingredients

3 cups rolled oats
1/2 cup almonds
1/2 cup pecans
1/4 cup sesame seeds
1/2 t cinnamon
1/4 to 1/2 t nutmeg
2 4-oz. jars baby food prunes or baby food applesauce
1/2 cup apple juice
1/3 cup oil
2 t vanilla

Method

1) Preheat oven to 300 degrees.
2) Grease a 15 x10 x 2 inch baking sheet.
3) Stir together the oats, almonds, pecans, sesame seeds, cinnamon and nutmeg.
4) Stir together the prunes (or applesauce), apple juice, oil and vanilla.
5) Add the liquid to the oat mixture and mix well.
6) Spread on baking sheet. Bake for 1 hour, stirring every 15 minutes. Cool completely and store in airtight containers or Ziploc bags.

Kasha Porridge

Ingredients

1 cup cooked kasha

1 apple, diced

2 T almond or cashew butter

1 t cinnamon

Method

1) Combine warm kasha and apple in a breakfast bowl.

2) In a separate bowl mix nut butter with 2 tablespoons of water. Blend with fork until creamy.

3) Pour over kasha and apples, sprinkle with cinnamon.

No Oat Oatmeal

Ingredients

1 small handful of walnuts
1 small handful of pecans
2 T ground flax seed
1/2–1 t ground cinnamon
1 pinch of ground nutmeg
1 pinch ground ginger
1 T almond butter
1 banana, mashed
3 eggs
1/4 cup unsweetened almond milk
2 t pumpkin seeds
1 handful of goji berries or fresh berries

Method

1) Add walnuts, pecans, flax seed and spices to a food processor and pulse it down to a course grain. Set aside.

2) Whisk together eggs and almond milk until the consistency thickens a little bit into a loose custard.

3) Thoroughly blend together the mashed banana and almond butter and add it to the custard, mixing well.

4) Stir in the nut mixture.

5) Microwave or gently warm on the stove until the "no-oatmeal" reaches your desired consistency.

6) Sprinkle pumpkin seeds and berries on top. Add more almond milk if you want.

Oatmeal Topping

Method

Mix 1 T peanut butter, 1/2 cup soy, rice or nut milk, a few drops of vanilla and a half of a banana in the food processor. Pour over cooked oatmeal.

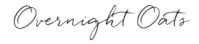

Overnight Oats

Ingredients

1 cup rolled oats
1/4 cup dried fruit (such as blueberries, raisins, cranberries, currants)
1/4 cup flax or sunflower seeds
Water

Method

1) The night before, place all ingredients in a bowl, then fill about 1/2 inch above oats with water.
2) Cover.
3) Place in a cool, dry place overnight.
4) In the morning, warm with a bit of water on the stove or eat at room temperature.

Variations:

In the morning you can heat up a cup of soy or rice milk to serve with oats and/or cut up fresh fruit to mix in.
Also try pumpkin seeds or chopped nuts to add variety.
Note: This is a great breakfast to bring along with you on the road. In a plastic container, pre-mix oats with your favorite toppings, add water to soak the oats, and take them with you.

Pumpkin, Buckwheat and Blueberry Porridge

Ingredients

2-1/2 cups milk (nut, rice or oat)
Dash of cinnamon
Dash of freshly ground nutmeg
Dash of dried lemon peel
Dash salt
Splash of maple flavoring (sugar and alcohol free)
1 T butter
1 jar baby-food pumpkin
1/2 cup cream of buckwheat
1/2 cup frozen blueberries

Method

1) Combine the first 8 ingredients in saucepan and cook over medium heat, bringing to a boil, stirring constantly.
2) Slowly stir in the Cream of Buckwheat and cook on medium-low heat about 8 minutes, stirring often.
3) Add blueberries, cover and let stand another 5 minutes. Stir to blend.

Quinoa with Dried Fruit and Nuts

Method

1) Prepare a batch of quinoa the night before (or save some leftovers from dinner).

   1 cup quinoa (rinse and drain)

   2 cups water

   Boil quinoa for 18 - 20 minutes and fluff with a fork. Refrigerate.

2) In the morning warm the quinoa on the stove with some almond, coconut or rice milk.

3) Add cinnamon, dried fruits (such as raisins, cranberries, cherries, mangos, apricots) and nuts or seeds of choice (sunflower, sesame, pumpkin, hemp, flax, chia, walnuts, almonds, pecans, hazelnuts).

Quinoa with Goji Berries, Macadamias and Vanilla

Ingredients

1 cup plain or red quinoa, rinsed well
2 cups water
1/4 cup almonds or macadamia nuts, roughly chopped
1/4 cup goji berries
1 vanilla pod, split and seeds scraped
2 t chia seeds
1 t ground ginger
Pinch cinnamon
1 lime, juice only
Yogurt for serving, if desired

Method

1) Cook the quinoa in 2 cups of water until boiling. Cover and simmer for 15 minutes.
2) Transfer cooked quinoa to a mixing bowl.
3) Add goji berries, macadamia nuts, vanilla seeds, chia, ginger and cinnamon.
4) Spoon into serving bowls.
5) Add a squeeze of lime and your favorite yogurt.

Quinoa Porridge with Carrots and Squash

Quinoa is gluten free and easily digestible. This protein-packed nutritional powerhouse is also high in magnesium, phosphorus, and iron. Start your day on the right note and enjoy the benefits of a steady flow of energy.

Ingredients
2 cups water
1 cup quinoa
¼ cup diced squash
¼ cup thinly sliced carrot rounds
¼ cup raisins
¼ cup walnuts
¼ cup sesame seeds
¼ cup plant-based milk (coconut, almond, hemp)

Method
1) Rinse quinoa well with cool water in a fine mesh strainer until the water runs clear.

2) Bring 2 cups of water to a boil. Add quinoa to boiling water. Reduce heat to a light boil and simmer for 20 minutes.

3) While cooking, add squash, carrots, raisins, walnuts, and sesame seeds. Add plant-based milk to desired consistency.

Quinoa Porridge with Nuts, Seeds and Fruit

Ingredients

1 cup cooked quinoa

2 T sunflower seeds, pumpkin seeds, or chopped walnuts

2 T raisins

2 T chopped dried apricots (substitute dried cranberries, currants, blueberries, chopped figs or dates as you like)

1/4 t salt

1/2 t cinnamon

1 cup almond, hemp or soy milk, flavored or plain - add more as needed

Method

1) Combine all ingredients in a two quart saucepan.

2) Heat on medium-low, stirring, until the quinoa has soaked up the liquid, and the dried fruit has plumped up nicely.

3) Add more milk if needed for consistency.

Quinoa Pumpkin Pie Spice Porridge

Ingredients

1/2 cup of quinoa – soaked and rinsed.

1 cup of almond milk blended with 2 dates for sweetness

½ t pumpkin pie spice

Method

1) Place almond milk and rinsed quinoa in a pot and bring to a boil, then simmer until the liquid is absorbed.

2) Stir in the pumpkin pie spice and enjoy warm or cold.
   Add some baked apple as a topping, if desired.

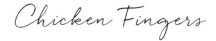

Chicken Fingers

Ingredients

½ cup whole grain bread crumbs (toast and process to crumbs bread of your choice) or ½ cup finely chopped pecans

1/8 t salt

1/8 t garlic powder

12 ounces boneless, skinless chicken breast cut into 1" x 3" strips

1 egg lightly beaten or 2 T milk

Method

1) Preheat oven to 400°F.

2) Mix crumbs, salt and pepper in bowl. Dip the chicken pieces first in either milk or egg and then dip them in the breadcrumbs to coat. Place chicken on an ungreased cookie sheet (or place on parchment paper for easier cleanup).

3) Bake 7-9 minutes until cooked through.

Lentil Stew for Breakfast

Ingredients

1 pound lentils

1 cup tomato sauce or several fresh tomatoes, chopped

4 cups chopped vegetables such as carrots, celery, onions, zucchini and / or parsnips

1 T broth base (such as Organic Better N Bullion)

2 T curry paste

1 cup salsa

Salt to taste

Method

1) Rinse lentils to remove stones or bad beans.

2) In a large pot, cook lentils in water plus one inch to cover.

3) While simmering, add tomato sauce or several chopped fresh tomatoes, and chopped vegetables.

4) Add broth base and water or broth as needed so lentils do not dry out.

5) Simmer until lentils are tender. Pink lentils take 20 minutes or so; green lentils may take up to an hour. (You can reduce cooking time by soaking overnight first.)

For additional flavor, add curry paste and/or salsa during the simmering.

Super Simple Turkey Chili

Method

1) Place enough olive oil in a soup pot to coat the bottom. On medium heat, brown 1½ pounds of ground turkey.

2) Add two cans of drained kidney or preferred beans

3) Add one small jar of salsa and one small jar of tomato sauce after reading the labels to make sure there is no form of sugar or corn syrup in them.

4) Add a tablespoon of chili powder, or to taste.

5) Add salt to taste, if it is not restricted for you.

6) Let it simmer until the water steams off and it is the consistency you like, about ½ hour.

Turkey Bacon and Kale

Ingredients

1 bunch of kale
4 strips of turkey bacon

Method

1) Slice turkey bacon into bite size pieces.
2) Place in pan and cook for a few minutes.
3) Chop kale, keeping the stems separate.
4) Add chopped stems to pan and cook for 1-2 minutes. Then add the rest of the kale, mix well with turkey bacon.
5) Add 1-2 tablespoons of water, cover and allow to cook for 3-4 minutes.
6) Remove cover, allow water to evaporate.
7) Add 1/2 of a raw grated carrot on top or sprinkle with sesame seeds and serve.

Turkey Sausage "Pancake"

Method

1) Take 1 lb of lean ground turkey and put it in a nonstick skillet. Mash it all flat into a big "pancake".

2) Sprinkle red Cajun seasoning on it to taste. Season with salt to taste.

3) Let the whole thing brown awhile on medium heat, flip, and cook until done.

Bacon and Egg Cupcakes

Method

1) Line muffin tins with bacon or ham.
2) Crack an egg in and bake at 375 degrees for about 10-12 minutes.
3) Sprinkle with feta cheese or chives.

Basic No-Recipe Frittata

Method

1) Put a little oil and butter in the skillet on top of the stove.

2) Overlap thinly sliced potatoes with the skin left on to make a thin layer and let it cook (without moving the potatoes around) until they start turning translucent.

3) Scatter some leftover veggies and shredded cheese over the potatoes (whatever you have on hand for both).

4) Pour beaten eggs over all and put it in the oven to finish cooking.

Breakfast Pie

Method

1) Cook some turkey sausage, crumbling it up during cooking. Put this in a pie pan to be the "crust".

2) Lightly brown some green pepper and onion and add it to the pie.

3) Add a layer of grated cheese.

4) Beat 6 eggs and a little milk and pour it into the pie.

5) Add some salt and paprika and bake it for about 30 minutes at 350 degrees Fahrenheit.

6) Add a small slice of tomato on top when it is done.

Egg, Sausage and Turnip Casserole

Turnips have the mildly earthy flavor that most root vegetables share and just a hint of sweetness.

Ingredients

1 pound ground breakfast sausage or other ground meat
3 turnips, peeled and grated (a food processor works well for this)
4 eggs, beaten
3 scallions, chopped

Method

1) Sauté sausage, breaking it up into small pieces with a spoon or spatula, until almost cooked through.
2) Mix the sausage with the rest of the ingredients.
3) Spoon into an 8×8 baking pan.
4) When ready to cook, heat oven to 400 degrees. Bake for 45 minutes then cover the pan and bake for 25 minutes more. Let cool 15-20 minutes so the casserole sets before cutting into it.

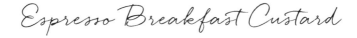

Espresso Breakfast Custard

Ingredients

2 1/2 cups milk (I used oat milk)

2 shots (1/2 cup) decaf espresso

3/4 cup nonfat dry milk

3 eggs

Cinnamon

Method

1) Preheat oven to 350° F.

2) In a saucepan, combine milk, espresso and dry milk. Place over medium heat and bring to a boil, stirring constantly to dissolve dry milk.

3) In a small bowl, beat eggs lightly. Add cinnamon to taste and then stir into heated milk very slowly (so you don't "cook" the eggs).

4) Pour into buttered custard cups, place in a shallow pan of hot water.

5) Bake for 40-45 minutes.

6) Sprinkle with slivered almonds just before eating to add a little more protein.

Frittata Muffins with Caramelized Onions, Kale and Golden Raisins

Ingredients

2 T butter or coconut oil, plus extra for muffin pan
1 onion, sliced or diced
1 t fresh (or dried) thyme
1/2 bunch kale, about 12 leaves, de-stem, chiffonade (slice thinly)
3 T Golden raisins
1/2 t kelp granules
1/2 t Celtic sea salt
9 eggs
3 T sour cream
1/2 cup cheddar cheese, grated

Method

1) Preheat oven to 350 degrees F. Grease muffin pan, set aside.
2) Melt butter in saucepan over medium-heat.
3) Prep onion, cut into thin slices or dice.
4) Add onion and thyme to the saucepan, stir occasionally.
5) Cook for about 15 minutes or until light golden brown/caramelized.
6) While onions are cooking, prep kale, de-stem and chiffonade or cut into small chunks.
7) When onions are caramelized, add kale, raisins, kelp granules and salt to the saucepan. Stir to combine, cook about 5 minutes.
8) Crack all eggs into a large mixing bowl. Break yolks with a whisk and stir to combine until egg mixture is yellow. Add sour cream and grated cheese, whisk to combine. Set aside.
9) Add about 1 1/2 teaspoons of onion-kale filling to each muffin hole.
10) Top onion-kale filling with about 3-4 tablespoons egg mixture (about 3/4 full).
11) Place muffin pan in oven and bake for about 25-30 minutes or until puffed and slightly golden brown on top.
12) Let cool in muffin pan for about 2-3 minutes before removing from pan to a cooling rack.

Frittatas

Frittatas, or Italian omelets, are a bit easier to make than omelets, though the techniques are similar. In addition to providing 5.5 grams of protein each, eggs are a valuable source of choline. Choline, found in egg yolks, is a micro-nutrient vital for optimum brain health, nerve signaling, cholesterol transport, energy metabolism and maintenance of cell membranes.

Ingredients

5 eggs
2 T grated Parmesan cheese
1 clove garlic, finely chopped
1/4 cup chopped onion
1 T olive oil
1 t Italian seasoning
1/2 t freshly ground black pepper
1/2 t salt
1/4 cup sliced mushrooms
1/2 cup sliced zucchini
1/2 cup asparagus, coarse ends removed, spears cut into 2-inch pieces
2 T grated cheddar cheese

Garnish

1 avocado, cut into wedges
1 tomato, cut into wedges

Method

1) Preheat broiler.
2) Lightly beat eggs and Parmesan cheese in a bowl.
3) Put the garlic, onions, and olive oil in an ovenproof sauté pan and cook over medium heat until the onions become limp. Add the spices. Add the mushrooms, zucchini, and asparagus and sauté until the onions are limp and transparent, about 2 1/2 to 3 minutes.
4) Pour the egg batter over the vegetables, shaking the pan to keep the eggs from sticking to the bottom. Loosen the edges of the omelet with a spatula and tilt the pan so that the uncooked part runs around the pan. Just before the eggs are about to set, sprinkle the grated cheddar

cheese on top and remove from the heat.

5) Put the pan under the broiler on the highest shelf until the top becomes brown, about 2 minutes. Slide the frittata onto a platter and cut into wedges. Garnish with avocado and tomato wedges. Serve immediately.

Italian Eggs

Method

1) Take 2 eggs and break them into a bowl.

2) Add 2 T water and blend well.

3) Add salt, pepper, a pinch of crushed fennel, crushed basil, a fresh mushroom diced small, a couple of green olives (sliced), a green onion (diced), and shredded cheddar or feta cheese.

4) Scramble in 2 teaspoons olive oil in a non-stick pan on medium heat.

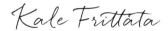

Kale Frittata

Ingredients

1 T olive oil
2 T finely chopped onion
1/2 cup or more finely chopped red cabbage
1 cup finely chopped kale
1 finely chopped red or yellow pepper
6 beaten eggs
A sprinkle of dried or fresh herbs (like oregano or basil)
Sausage to serve on the side

Method

1) Preheat broiler.
2) Warm olive oil in an ovenproof pan and sauté onions until they begin to soften.
3) Add cabbage and sauté about three minutes then add kale and peppers.
5) Continue to sauté until kale wilts.
6) Add salt and pepper to taste.
7) Pour in eggs, stir quickly then let cook until it just barely begins to set.
8) Put the frittata under a broiler until the top is golden and the eggs are cooked through, 3–5 minutes.

Millet Tofu Patties

Ingredients

1/2 block of tofu
1 cup millet
1 cup mustard greens chopped
1 medium onion, finely chopped
1 clove garlic, minced
1 tablespoon tamari
3 cups water or veggie stock, boiled
Dash of cayenne pepper

Method

1) In a saucepan, sauté onions and garlic in a dash of olive oil for 3 minutes.

2) Stir in millet grains, frying until they are lightly colored.

3) Pour boiling water over millet, onions, garlic and cover.

4) Cook on medium-low for 20-30 minutes until liquid is evaporated.

5) Blend millet, mustard greens, tamari, cayenne and tofu in blender.

6) Spread out on baking sheet about 2/3 of an inch thick and chill thoroughly.

7) Cut into 8 flat cakes.

8) Heat broiler or toaster oven.

9) Broil or toast on each side until golden brown.

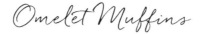

Ingredients

6 eggs

1/4 – 1/2 cup cooked meat, cut or crumbled into small pieces

1/2 cup diced vegetables

1/4 t salt

1/8 t ground pepper

1/8 cup mayonnaise

1/8 cup water

Optional Ingredient Idea: Make a Mexican Omelet Muffin by adding 1/4 cup shredded cheese, onions, and lightly drained salsa to the eggs.

Method

1) Preheat oven to 350°F.
2) Generously grease 6 muffin tins with butter or coconut oil or for easier removal line with paper baking cups. The baking cups also help the muffins hold their shape.
3) In a bowl, beat the eggs.
4) Add meat, vegetables, salt, ground pepper, and any other ingredients and stir to combine. Spoon or scoop into the muffin cups.
5) Bake for 18–20 minutes until a knife inserted into the center of a muffin/omelet comes out almost clean.
6) Remove the omelets from the muffin cups and serve, or cool completely and store for another day.

Portobello and Asparagus Egg Strata

Ingredients

1 T extra virgin olive oil
1 1/2 cups chopped yellow onion
1/4 t dried thyme
3 cloves garlic, finely chopped
1 cup Portobello mushrooms, thinly sliced
1/2 pound asparagus, trimmed and cut into 1-inch lengths
1 t salt
8 eggs
1 cup milk
2 T Dijon mustard
3 T chopped parsley
Black pepper to taste
5 cups (1-inch) cubes sourdough bread
4 ounces herb or plain goat cheese, crumbled

Method

1) Heat oil in a large skillet over medium heat. Add onions and thyme and cook until softened, about 4 minutes. Add garlic, mushrooms, asparagus and 1/2 teaspoon of the salt and cook 5 more minutes longer. Set aside.

2) Meanwhile, whisk together eggs, milk, mustard, parsley, pepper and remaining 1/2 teaspoon salt in a large bowl. Set aside.

3) Spread half of the bread over the bottom of a lightly greased 9-x13-inch baking dish. Top with half of the mushroom mixture and a third of the goat cheese. Layer with remaining bread and mushroom mixture, and pour egg mixture evenly over the top. Cover strata and chill overnight.

4) Preheat oven to 375°F. Remove strata from refrigerator and bring to room temperature while the oven heats. Sprinkle remaining two-thirds goat cheese over the top and bake until firm in the center and golden brown on top, about 45 minutes. Let rest 10 minutes before serving.

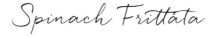
Spinach Frittata

Ingredients

1 lb spinach leaves (about 2 bunches), cleaned, chopped
1 T olive oil
1 medium onion, chopped (about 1 cup)
1 large clove garlic, minced
9 large eggs
2 T milk
1/3 cup grated Parmesan cheese
Sun-dried tomatoes, about 2 Tbsp chopped
Salt and freshly ground pepper to taste
3 oz. goat cheese

Method

1) Preheat oven to 400°F.

2) Cook spinach in 1/4 cup of water in a covered saucepan until just wilted, a couple minutes. Drain water and set aside.

3) In a mixing bowl, whisk together eggs, milk, and Parmesan cheese. Add in chopped sun-dried tomatoes, and sprinkle with salt and pepper. Set aside.

4) Sauté onions in olive oil in an oven-proof, stick-free skillet, until translucent, about 4-5 minutes on medium heat. Add garlic and cook a minute further. Add cooked spinach and mix in with onions and garlic.

5) Spread out spinach mixture evenly on bottom of skillet. Pour egg mixture over spinach mixture. Use a spatula to lift up the spinach mixture along the sides of the pan to let egg mixture flow underneath.

6) Sprinkle bits of goat cheese over the top of the frittata mixture. When the mixture is about half set, put the whole pan in the oven. Bake for 13-15 minutes, until frittata is puffy and golden. Remove from oven with oven mitts and let cool for several minutes.

Two-Minute Egg Soufflé

Ingredients

1 egg(s)
2 egg white(s)
1 T salsa

Method

1) Spray a small microwave-safe bowl with oil spray.

2) Crack egg and egg whites into the bowl and whip together with a fork.

3) Add one heaping tablespoon of salsa and a squirt of hot sauce, if desired.

4) Mix well.

5) Microwave for 2 minutes, or until egg is just cooked through.

Vegetable Quiche with Potato Crust

Ingredients

1/2 cup water
1/4 cup sun-dried tomatoes
1/2 pound asparagus (about 2 cups chopped) or broccoli florets
1/2 medium onion, chopped
2 cloves garlic, sliced
2 T extra-virgin olive oil
1 carrot, cut in small cubes (about 1 cup)
5 mushrooms, sliced
1 T chopped fresh basil, or 1 teaspoon dried
1 T chopped fresh parsley
1/8 t chili flakes
1/8 t freshly grated nutmeg
1/2 t salt
1 t freshly ground black pepper
3 small red potatoes, washed and thinly sliced
1/2 cup grated cheese, Pepper Jack or Swiss
1/4 cup milk
1/2 cup sour cream
6 eggs
1 medium tomato, sliced (seeds squeezed out)
3 T freshly grated Parmesan cheese

Method

1) Preheat oven to 375° F.

2) Boil the water, pour over the sun-dried tomatoes, and allow to soak for about 15 minutes until they become soft and plump. Strain off any remaining liquid, and coarsely chop.

3) Cut off about 1 inch of the coarse ends of the asparagus stalks and discard. Cut the remaining stalks into about 6 pieces or chop coarsely. (If you are using broccoli, cut into florets.)

4) Blanch the asparagus by boiling it in a medium pot of water for 2 minutes or less. Asparagus should be bright green and firm to the bite. Drain, rinse the asparagus in cold water, and drain again in a colander.

5) Sauté the onions and the garlic in the olive oil over low heat until the onions are transparent, approximately 10 minutes. Add the carrots, mushrooms, basil, parsley, chili flakes, nutmeg, salt and pepper and continue to cook for 5 more minutes. Remove from the heat.

6) Lightly grease the bottom and sides of a 9-inch pie pan. Line the bottom with the potato slices, overlapping them slightly.

7) Whisk together the cheese, milk, sun-dried tomatoes, sour cream and the eggs in a large bowl. Mix in the sautéed vegetables and the blanched asparagus, coating everything with the cheese, milk and egg liquid, then pour into the potato-lined pie pan. Arrange the tomato slices on top and sprinkle with Parmesan cheese.

8) Bake for 1 hour, covering after 45 minutes if top browns. Completely baked quiche should be very firm.

Let cool 15 minutes before slicing and serving.

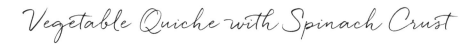

Vegetable Quiche with Spinach Crust

Crust
6 cups fine chopped spinach
2 T Olive oil
1/4 cup fresh chopped basil
2 cloves garlic, minced
3/4 cup chopped sunflower seeds

Filling
1 cup chopped asparagus
1 cup cooking greens of choice (spinach, kale, collards, dandelion greens)
½ cup chopped portabella mushrooms
6-8 eggs
2 T nutritional yeast
¾ cup almond, or hemp milk
Herbs of choice (dill, basil, cilantro, thyme- all good in here)
Salt and pepper

Method
Preheat oven to 350º F.

Crust
1) In a medium size sauté pan, sauté garlic and spinach in olive oil over medium heat for 2-3 minutes. Add in crushed sunflower seeds and basil. Stir well and cook together another 2-3 minutes.
2) Remove from heat and drain off any excess cooking liquid. Spoon into the bottom of your pie/baking pan and shape to cover bottom and edges.

Filling
1) Whisk together eggs and milk.
2) Stir in chopped vegetables.

Zucchini Ricotta Cheesecake

Ingredients

2 cups zucchini, unpeeled & grated
1 t fine grain sea salt
2 1/2 cups ricotta cheese
1/2 cup freshly shredded Parmesan cheese
2 shallots, chopped
2 cloves garlic, chopped
1/4 cup fresh dill, chopped
Zest of one lemon
2 large eggs, well beaten
1/3 cup goat cheese, crumbled
Drizzle of olive oil

Method

1) Preheat oven to 325F degrees, with racks the middle. Butter/oil a 7-inch spring form pan.

2) In a strainer, toss the shredded zucchini with the salt and let sit for ten minutes. Squeeze and press out as much moisture as you can. Set aside.

3) In the meantime, combine the ricotta cheese, Parmesan cheese, shallots, garlic, dill and lemon zest in a medium bowl. Stir in the eggs and continue mixing until well combined. Now stir in the shredded zucchini.

4) Fill the spring form pan with the ricotta mixture and place on a baking sheet. Place in the oven and bake for sixty minutes. If there is any moisture left on top of the cake at this point, carefully use a bit of paper towel to dab it off. Now sprinkle with the goat cheese and return to the oven for another 20 -30 minutes or until the goat cheese is melted and the cake barely jiggles in the center (it will set up more as it cools).

5) At this point, if the cake is baked and set, but the top isn't quite golden, put it under the broiler for about a minute to get more color on top. Remove from the oven and let cool five minutes, then release the cake from its pan. Cool completely, serve at room temperature drizzled with a bit of olive oil and a few sprigs of dill.

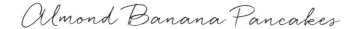

Almond Banana Pancakes

Ingredients

2 ripe bananas

1 egg

1 heaping T of almond butter

Method

1) Mash the bananas, add the egg and mix well.

2) Stir in the almond butter, adding more than a tablespoon if you want a more pancake-like texture.

3) Warm butter in a pan and pour batter into small pancakes.

4) Brown on each side and serve warm with a pat of butter, a scoop of nut butter or fresh berries.

Easy Egg and Oat Pancakes

Ingredients

2 eggs
3/4 cup milk or yogurt
1 cup oats
1 small apple, diced
Cinnamon and nutmeg to taste

Method

1) Beat the eggs, stir in milk or yogurt.
2) Add oats, apple, nutmeg and cinnamon.
3) Cook like a pancake.
4) Garnish with a little plain yogurt.

Oatmeal and Protein Pancakes

Method

In a blender, mix:
3 eggs
1/2 cup cottage cheese
1/2 cup oatmeal (uncooked)
1 t baking powder
1/2 t baking soda
1 t vanilla or 1 t maple flavoring

Blend until it's all mixed well. If it's too thick, add a little milk or cottage cheese.

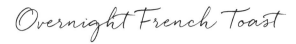

Overnight French Toast

Ingredients

4 T butter

10 slices of leftover whole grain bread (whole wheat, whole spelt, Ezekiel, brown rice, etc.)

7 eggs

1 ¾ cups milk (cow, soy, oat, almond)

3 T apple juice

1 T maple flavoring (sugar free)

1 ½ t vanilla flavoring (sugar free)

1/2 t salt

Protein Powder (as desired)

The night before:

Spread butter over the bottom of a large baking sheet with 1-inch high sides (jelly roll pan). Arrange bread slices on pan, making sure they do not overlap. Combine remaining ingredients in a blender and pour mixture evenly over slices of bread. Turn the slices to coat evenly. Cover with plastic wrap and refrigerate overnight.

In the morning:

Preheat oven to 400°F.

Place baking sheet in oven and bake for 10 minutes. Turn over slices of bread and continue baking until golden brown, about 5 minutes more.

Pumpkin Pancakes

Ingredients

1 1/4 c. whole oats ground with 1/4 c. protein powder until flour consistency

1 ½ t baking powder

½ t salt

1/2 t cinnamon

1/4 t ground cloves

1/4 t ginger

1 cup milk

1 T oil

1 egg

1/2 – 1 cups pumpkin

Method

1) Mix the wet ingredients together.

2) Stir the wet ingredients into the dry.

3) Cook in a lightly greased skillet/electric fry pan.

4) Serve with cream cheese or whipped cream (homemade with just a drop or two of vanilla.)

Sweet Potato Waffles (or Pancakes)

Ingredients

1/2 pound sweet potatoes, peeled, cooked and mashed (about 3/4 cup)
1 1/2 t oil
1 large egg white, lightly beaten
3/4 cup milk (cow, soy, oat)
1/2 cup brown rice flour
1 t baking powder
1/4 t salt (optional)

Method

1) Preheat waffle iron.

2) Combine the cooked sweet potato, oil, egg white and milk in a large bowl and beat until well blended. Add flour, baking powder and salt and beat until smooth.

3) Spray hot waffle iron with non-stick cooking spray. Cook waffles according to manufacturer's instructions using 3/4 c mix per waffle.

4) Serve with yogurt, fresh fruit, fruit compote or unsweetened apple sauce.

If making pancakes, heat griddle until a sprinkle of water dances on griddle. Drop 1/4 cup batter on griddle. Cook until bubbles form on surface (about 3 minutes). Flip and cook on other side until golden brown.

Both waffles and pancakes can be frozen and reheated later.

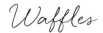

Waffles

Ingredients

1 cup oat flour
1 cup brown rice flour
½ cup protein powder
1 t baking soda
½ t cinnamon
½ t salt
2 cups oat milk
2 eggs
1/3 cup butter, melted and cooled

Method

1) In a bowl mix together oat flour, brown rice flour, protein powder, baking soda, cinnamon and salt.
2) In another bowl mix together oat milk, eggs and butter.
3) Add wet ingredients to dry and cook in waffle iron.

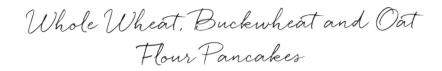

Whole Wheat, Buckwheat and Oat Flour Pancakes

Ingredients

1/2 cup whole wheat flour
1/4 cup buckwheat flour
1/4 cup oat flour
2 t baking powder
1/2 t salt
1 egg
3/4 milk
1/4 cup oil

Method

1) Mix the dry ingredients in a bowl.
2) Combine the egg, milk and oil.
3) Stir together until just moistened.
4) Cook on hot greased griddle (or pan).

For more flavor, you can add vanilla, a banana, an apple or chocolate or vanilla almond milk. You can top them with a berry compote made from frozen blueberries and a little fruit juice cooked on the stove.

Smoothie Basics

For an instant healthy makeover, just add a smoothie into your daily routine. Smoothies are a perfect opportunity to sneak in limitless amounts of vegetables, some fruit and even some protein.

Ice: Always start with a handful of ice at the bottom of the blender. Smoothies are meant to be cold, and putting the ice in first ensures the blender blades crush the cubes thoroughly.

Banana: Bananas add a creaminess and density to smoothies. Use ripe (even overly ripe) bananas because they will provide more natural sugars and flavor. Mangos are a good substitute.

Greens: Dark leafy greens give your smoothies their superpowers. Start with fresh baby spinach because of its mild flavor. Then work your way up to dandelion greens, kale, chard, collards, parsley and romaine lettuce.

Frozen fruit: Add a cup or two of frozen fruit like blueberries, strawberries, pineapple, acai, etc. Although fresh fruit is more than fine, frozen fruit is often less expensive, lasts longer, and provides a better frozen-treat texture.

Nut milk: Pour in about a cup of unsweetened nut milk like almond or hazelnut for healthy and delicious creaminess. Allergic to nuts? Try hemp milk, rice milk, or soymilk instead.

Superfoods and protein powders: Add in a few spoonfuls of protein powder, superfood powders, freeze-dried greens, etc.

Water: Top off your smoothie by pouring water into the full blender, just about an inch or two above the rest of the ingredients, so that it's easy to blend.

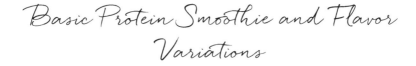

Basic Protein Smoothie and Flavor Variations

Basic Recipe

- 2 cups of milk, soymilk, almond milk or oat milk
- 2 T protein powder
- 2 T oatmeal (not instant)

Variations

- **Apple Crisp:** Add precooked oatmeal, red delicious apple, walnuts and ½ tsp cinnamon
- **Banana-Peanut Butter:** Use chocolate almond milk, oats, banana, and peanut (or almond) butter.
- **Berry:** Add frozen berries of your choice.
- **Chocolate:** Use chocolate almond milk.
- **Icy Espresso:** Add 1 shot decaf espresso, handful of almonds and ice.
- **Mocha:** Use part chocolate flavored almond milk and part decaf for your liquid.
- **Orange Dreamsicle:** Add ¼ cup frozen orange juice concentrate, 1/3 frozen banana and a handful of ice. Add some yogurt to give it a bit of tang.
- **Pina Colada:** Add pineapple and coconut.
- **Praline Shake:** Add banana, pecans and maple flavoring.
- **Pumpkin or Sweet Potato:** Add frozen sweet potato and/or pumpkin (freeze in ice-cube trays), vanilla / cinnamon / nutmeg / or pumpkin pie spice for flavoring.
- **Strawberry Cheesecake:** Add ricotta cheese, cream cheese and frozen strawberries.

Apple Crisp Smoothie

Ingredients
1 scoop protein powder
1/4 cup oatmeal
2 cups cold nut milk of your choice
1 sliced apple, skin on
2 t. walnuts
½ t. cinnamon

Banana Oat Smoothie

Ingredients
1 ripe banana
1/2 cup low-fat plain yogurt
1/2 cup skim milk
1/4 cup old-fashioned rolled oats
2 t flaxseeds
1 cup ice

Banana Peanut Butter Smoothie

Ingredients
1 ripe banana
1 cup low-fat milk
1/4 cup peanut butter
1/2 cup ice

Banana Spinach Smoothie

Ingredients

2 cups spinach
2 frozen bananas
1 1/2 cups unsweetened almond milk
1 T protein powder

Banana Superfood Green Smoothie

Ingredients

8 oz of nut milk
1 frozen banana
5-6 medium size fresh strawberries
1 T hemp seeds
1 T chia seeds
1 T maca
1 T protein powder
1 inch piece of vanilla bean or vanilla extract
2-4 Medjool dates (pitted)
Pinch of salt

Berry Almond Smoothie

Ingredients

1 frozen banana
1 cup frozen strawberries
1 cup frozen blueberries
2 T almond butter
1 T flax seed
2 cups unsweetened almond milk

Berry Tofu Smoothie

Ingredients

1/2 cup silken tofu
1 ripe banana
2 cups frozen mixed berries
1/2 cup fresh orange juice

Blackberry Cinnamon Smoothie

Ingredients

1 1/2 cups frozen blackberries
1/2 cup low-fat plain yogurt
1/2 cup low-fat buttermilk
1 T honey
1/8 t ground cinnamon

Blueberry Almond Butter Smoothie

Ingredients

1 ripe banana
1 1/2 cups frozen blueberries
1 T lemon juice
3 Ta lmond butter
2 T flaxseeds
3 dates (Medjool or Deglet), pitted
2 cups water

Blueberry Flax Smoothie

Ingredients

  1 ripe banana
  1 cup frozen blueberries
  1 cup low-fat plain yogurt
  4 t flaxseeds
  1 T honey

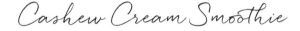

Cashew Cream Smoothie

Ingredients

  1 cup boiling water
  1 cup raw cashews
  1 cup ice
  1 vanilla bean, seeds scraped (reserve the bean itself for another use), or
  1 teaspoon pure vanilla extract
  1 T agave nectar

Method

1) Pour boiling water over cashews and let stand until softened, about 15 minutes.

2) Puree in a blender on high speed for 3 minutes until smooth.

3) Add ice and vanilla extract or seeds. Blend until smooth. Add agave nectar to taste.

Calcium Blaster

Recently I was diagnosed with osteoporosis. So I try to incorporate as much calcium as possible into my diet. This smoothie gives me almost 100% of the daily requirements of calcium ... for a normal person that is. I need about twice that, so this smoothie gets me half-way where I need to go each day!

It's simple to make in my NutriBullet, and it's easy to keep the ingredients on hand. I always have frozen collard greens in my freezer, and sometimes frozen bananas, too. I even pour almond milk into an ice cube tray and freeze it! You just can't have ALL of your ingredients frozen to begin with or your NutriBullet will just freeze up, too! If your collard greens are frozen it's best to use a fresh banana and vice versa.

Ingredients
1 cup frozen collard greens
2 cups unsweetened vanilla almond milk
1 banana
1 T raw cacao

Method
1) Put the collard greens in the large cup of a NutriBullet.
2) Add the banana, almond milk and cacao.
3) Blend.

Chocolate Almond Smoothie

Ingredients
1 ripe banana
1 cup low-fat milk
1/4 cup almond butter
1 scoop protein powder
2 T unsweetened cocoa powder
1/2 cup ice

Chocolate Avocado Smoothie

Avocado and chocolate make an incredibly indulgent combo. Here, their flavors blend with banana and other natural ingredients to create a uniquely delicious, creamy treat.

Ingredients
1 ripe avocado, peeled and pitted
2 T dark unsweetened cocoa powder
2 T agave nectar
1 frozen banana
1 cup ice
1 cup unsweetened almond milk
1 scoop protein powder

Chocolate Berry Superfood Smoothie

Ingredients

2 cups mixed frozen berries (blueberries, raspberries, blackberries)
1/2 cup goji berries
1/4 cup mulberries
3-4 T cacao powder
2 T acai powder
4 T hemp seeds
2 cups hemp milk
1 cup water
Handful ice

Chocolate Goodness Smoothie

Ingredients

Handful ice
1 banana
1 cup frozen blueberries
1 cup unsweetened hemp milk
1 scoop chocolate protein powder
1 t wheatgrass powder
2 T raw cacao powder
1 t mesquite powder
Stevia powder, to taste
2-3 cups water

Chocolate Raspberry Smoothie

Ingredients

Handful ice
1 banana
1 cup frozen blueberries
1 cup unsweetened hemp milk
1 scoop chocolate protein powder
1 t wheatgrass powder
2 T raw cacao powder
1 t mesquite powder
Stevia powder, to taste
2-3 cups water

Chocolate Almond Smoothie

Ingredients

1 large ripe banana, frozen
1 cup frozen raspberries
1 T cacao powder
3 dates, pitted and chopped
1 cup almond milk

Green Power Smoothie

Ingredients

1.5 cups almond milk (I like unsweetened vanilla)
1 banana
3 large kale leaves (or spinach or collard greens)
3 to 5 whole dates, pitted
1 T protein powder

Mango Banana Coconut Smoothie

Ingredients

- 2 cups mango chunks
- 2 frozen bananas
- 2 T shredded coconut
- 1 cup ice
- 1 1/4 cups almond milk
- 1 1/4 cups coconut milk
- 2 T protein powder

Mango Dessert Smoothie

Ingredients

- 2 heaping cups frozen mango chunks
- 1/2 cup hemp milk
- 1/2 cup water
- 1 scoop vanilla protein powder
- Touch of stevia, to taste (optional)
- 2 T shredded coconut (optional)

Method

Blend mangos, hemp milk, water, and protein powder together in a blender until completely smooth. If desired, boost sweetness with a touch of Stevia, to taste, and blend again. Serve in a bowl and top with shredded coconut. Serves 2.

Pumpkin, Kale, Cacao Protein Smoothie

Ingredients
1 scoop protein powder
½ cup berries (strawberries, blueberries and/or raspberries)
¼ cup pumpkin puree
1 t unsweetened cocoa powder
½ cup kale

Pumpkin Spice Smoothie

Pumpkin is high in antioxidants and a great source of energy to keep you fueled throughout the day. This smoothie is also an excellent precursor to winter with both the warming and anti-inflammatory properties of cinnamon, ginger and nutmeg.

Ingredients
½ cup pureed pumpkin (fresh or canned)
1 cup almond milk
1 banana, sliced and frozen ahead of time
1 carrot (optional)
1 scoop vanilla protein powder
½ t vanilla extract or powdered vanilla bean
1 sliver fresh ginger root
Sprinkle nutmeg and cinnamon to taste

Strawberry Smoothie

Ingredients
1 ripe banana
1 1/2 cups frozen strawberries (10-oz. package)
3/4 cup plain low-fat yogurt
2 T honey

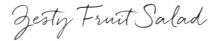

Zesty Fruit Salad

Ingredients
2 cup blueberries
3-4 nectarines, sliced
1 cup sliced strawberries
2 T balsamic vinegar
¼ t black pepper.

Method
1) Mix vinegar and pepper in a small bowl.
2) Pour over cut fruit and stir to coat.
3) Serve cold.

Black Bean and Quinoa Salad

Ingredients

2 cups black beans, cooked (use canned beans if you're short on time)
1 cup quinoa, rinsed
2 cups water
1 red onion, peeled and minced
1 red pepper, deseeded and diced small
12 ounces, cooked chicken breast, shredded (drag a fork through cooked chicken breast to create shredded pieces)
1/4 cup cilantro
Juice of 2 limes
2 T red wine vinegar
1 T brown rice syrup
1/3 cup olive oil
1 t cumin
Sea salt to taste

Method

1) Bring quinoa and water to a boil. Cover and simmer on low for 12-15 minutes or until all the water is absorbed.

2) In a large bowl, combine cooked quinoa with beans, red onion, red pepper, cooked shredded chicken, and cilantro.

3) Whisk together lime juice, red wine vinegar, rice malt syrup, olive oil. cumin and sea salt.

4) Pour dressing onto black bean and quinoa salad and mix thoroughly.

Black Bean Salsa

Ingredients
3 large ripe tomatoes
1 cup black beans
¾ cup cooked corn kernels
1/4 cup chopped fresh cilantro
½ large red onion, minced
1 T minced hot pepper of choice (optional)
2 cloves garlic, minced
1 tbsp olive oil
3 Tbsp apple cider vinegar

Method
1) In a small skillet, heat olive oil and then add in garlic and onions. Sauté for 3-4 minutes over medium heat and transfer to a large mixing bowl.

2) Chop tomatoes to desired chunk size. You can take 1cup of tomato and puree it for a "soupy" salsa or leave all in chunks for a chunkier version.

3) Toss in all of your remaining ingredients and mix wel l to blend.

Carrot Ginger Soup

Ingredients

4 cups chopped carrots
6 cups vegetable stock
1 medium onion, minced
2 inch nub ginger root, peeled and grated
Salt to taste
Dash nutmeg
Chopped fresh parsley, dill, or cilantro

Method

1) Put carrots, ginger, and onion in pot with stock. Bring to boil, cover, reduce heat and simmer 20-25 minutes.

2) Remove from heat and put everything in a blender or food processor to puree. Serve hot topped with herbs.

Chickpea, Edamame and Carrot Salad

Ingredients

1 can (15 ounces) chickpeas or garbanzo beans, rinsed
3/4 cup edamame (thaw if frozen)
1/4 cup red bell pepper, finely chopped
1/4 cup green pepper, finely chopped
1/3 cup carrot, finely chopped
1/3 cup dried cranberries (unsweetened)
2 T olive oil
1/4 cup balsamic vinegar
1/2 t sea salt
1-2 cloves garlic, minced
1/2 t cumin
1 t Italian seasoning
1/4 t rosemary
black pepper to taste

Method

1) Mix together oil, vinegar, sea salt, garlic, cumin, Italian seasoning, rosemary and black pepper

2) In a large bowl mix together the chickpeas, edamame, peppers, carrots and cranberries.

3) Toss with dressing and stir to evenly coat.

4) Refrigerate salad for at least an hour before serving to let flavors set in.

Green Bean and Almond Salad

Ingredients

2 pounds of fresh beans, snapped and steamed.
½ cup chopped raw almonds (roasted is ok too if you can't find raw)
2 T fresh minced dill
1 T olive oil
2 T lemon juice
Salt and pepper

Method

1) After beans are steamed and cooled, toss with all remaining ingredients.
2) Allow to marinate for 15 minutes to overnight.

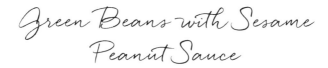

Green Beans with Sesame Peanut Sauce

Ingredients

3 cup fresh beans with ends cut off
1/4cup nut butter (peanut, almond, cashew, or sun butter)
2 T sesame oil
2 T rice vinegar
3 t wheat free tamari
1 inch nub ginger root, grated

Method

1) Steam beans for 2-3 minutes.
2) Combine all other ingredients in a small bowl and whisk.
3) Remove beans from heat and rinse in cold water.
4) Toss beans with sauce and serve.

Roasted Broccoli

Method

1) Preheat oven to 375°

2) Chop a head of broccoli. Rinse, and make sure it is completely dry.

3) Mince 2-3 cloves of garlic

4) Put broccoli, garlic, 2 Tolive oil, and a few shakes of salt and pepper in a baggie.

5) Shake.

6) Spread out on baking sheet, place on top rack, and bake for about 30 minutes. Broccoli will be crunchy and delicious!

Roasted Sweet Potato, Corn and Cannellini Bean Salad

Ingredients
2 cups small diced sweet potatoes
2 – 3 ears of corn
1 ½ cups cooked or canned cannellini beans
¼ cup small diced red onion
½ t salt
Black pepper to taste
½ t smoked paprika
¼ cup olive oil
2 T lime juice
2 T chopped cilantro

Method
1) Remove corn from the cob.
2) Toss corn and yams separately each with 1 tablespoon of the olive oil, a pinch of the salt, black pepper to taste, and half each of the paprika.
3) Place in a baking pan and bake at 450 degrees for 10–12 minutes or until the vegetables are tender and a little browned. Remove from oven and let cool.
4) Toss the corn and yams with the cannellini beans, red onion, and cilantro.
5) Combine the remaining olive oil, lime juice, salt and paprika and toss into vegetables.
6) Adjust seasoning to taste. Serve.

Crock Pot Spaghetti Squash

One of the advantages of cooking an entire spaghetti squash in your crock pot is that you don't have to slice it in half in its raw state … always such a scary adventure.

The other advantage is coming home to a cooked squash!

Method

1) Wash squash.
2) Poke several times with a fork or knife to avoid an exploding squash.
3) Place in crock pot with 1.5 cups water.
4) Cover and cook on low 6- 9 hours, depending on the size of the squash.
5) Remove and cool 30 minutes.
6) Slice carefully and remove seeds.
7) Shred insides with a fork.
8) Season and serve.

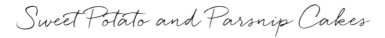

Ingredients

2 baked sweet potatoes
4 baked parsnips
1 large onion, chopped
2 cloves garlic, minced
1 egg
¼ t salt

Method

1) Bake sweet potatoes and parsnips in a covered casserole dish at 375 for about 30-45 minutes.

2) Remove from heat and reduce oven heat to 325.

3) Put parsnip and "meat" of sweet potato into a food processor or blender and mix well. Remove and place in bowl.

4) Add all remaining ingredients and stir well.

5) Form into patties and place on lightly oiled baking sheet in oven.

6) Bake for 25 minutes. Remove from oven and enjoy.

Sweet Potato "Sandwiches"

Method

1) Slice 4 to 6 sweet potato rounds (depending on size) to your desired thickness.

2) Add a teaspoon or two of safflower oil to a stovetop pan and throw the sweet potatoes in until they crisp up (about 5 to 10 minutes).

3) Of if you're really short on time, skip the pan approach altogether and stick the slices in the microwave for two minutes to soften them.

4) Variation 1: Goat Cheese. CombE goat cheese crumbles (or even cream cheese or vegan cheese such as Daiya) with pomegranate seeds and crushed walnuts. Spread the mixture on one sweet potato round, top with spinach, and stack another round on top!

5) Variation 2: Coat your sweet potatoes with black beans that you've cooked on the stove and mashed. Spread this in a thin layer and top with slices of avocado and tomato, plus some sprigs of cilantro (dried works, too!). Finish it off with a small dollop of tofu sour cream.

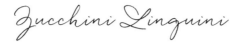

Ingredients

1 large zucchini
1 large yellow squash
1 cup cherry or plum tomatoes
4 cloves garlic, minced
1/4cup fresh basil
1/4cup olive oil
3 cups fresh leaf spinach

Method

1) Slice zucchini and yellow squash in half and remove seeds from center. Proceed to slice squash into long thin strips, like linguini. Steam until soft, about 3-5 minutes. Start with the yellow squash and steam that for an extra couple of minutes because the skin is harder and needs a little more cook time.

2) In the meantime, sauté garlic over medium heat in 2 T of the olive oil for about 4 minutes, until browned. Set aside.

3) In a blender or food processor, puree remaining oil with the basil and garlic.

4) Fine chop spinach and cut tomatoes in half.

5) When squash is soft, remove from heat. Toss with garlic, olive oil/ba sil/garlic combination. Gently toss in spinach and tomatoes.

6) Serve warm.

Basic Salad Dressing Formula and Tips

Basic Salad Dressing Formula:

3 parts oil	Avocado Grapeseed Olive Peanut Pumpkin Seed Sesame Walnut
1 part vinegar or acidic juice	Balsamic Champagne Rice Lemon Orange
And a few flavor boosters!	Fresh Herbs Garlic Ginger Honey Mustard Shallots Soy Sauce Tahini

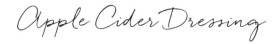

Apple Cider Dressing

Ingredients

¾ cup vegetable stock
2 T corn starch or arrowroot
¼ cup apple cider vinegar
2 t Dijon mustard
1 T shallot
2 T fresh herbs (basil, thyme and oregano mixed)
1 T honey
2 T olive oil

Method

1) Mix ¼ cup cold vegetable stock with 2 T corn starch or arrowroot. Bring ½ cup vegetable stock to a boil, whisk in cold vegetable stock and cornstarch mixture. Chill until completely cooled and jelled.

2) Purée all ingredients except olive oil.

3) Slowly add in olive oil to emulsify.

Balsamic Vinaigrette

Ingredients

1⅓ cups virgin olive oil
⅔ cup balsamic vinegar
1 t chili pepper flakes
1 T finely minced garlic
½ t salt (optional)
2 T parsley, minced
2 T fresh basil, chopped fine

Method

Combine all ingredients.

Light Balsamic Dressing

Ingredients

1/2 cup balsamic vinegar
3 T extra-virgin olive oil
1/4 cup water
1 T Dijon mustard*
1 t honey
1 t garlic powder

Method

Combine all ingredients in a jar or container with a screw-on lid. Shake vigorously until everything is well combined.

Basil Balsamic

Ingredients

1/2 cup fresh basil leaves
1/3 cup balsamic vinegar
1/3 cup shallots, chopped
1/4 cup water
1 T olive oil

Method

Put everything in a blender and process until smooth.

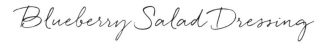

Blueberry Salad Dressing

Ingredients
½ cup frozen blueberries
¾ cup flax oil
1/3 cup apple cider vinegar
Dash of sea salt
1 T honey

Method
1) Pulse in blender very briefly.
2) Put in airtight container and store in fridge.

Caesar Salad Dressing

Ingredients
1 T lemon juice
2 T mayonnaise
1/2 cup extra-virgin olive oil
6 garlic cloves, minced
1 T Dijon mustard
Minced anchovy fillets
Sea salt and freshly ground black pepper to taste

Method
1) Using a blender, process the lemon juice, garlic and mustard.
2) Add the mayonnaise and blend again.
3) Slowly add the olive oil while the blender is in motion.
4) Use a spatula to scrape the dressing into a bowl.
5) Season with salt and pepper.
6) Add some more lemon juice to taste.
7) Add minced anchovy fillets to taste..

No Egg Caesar Salad Dressing

Ingredients
1½ T garlic, minced
4½ T lemon juice
3 filets anchovies
2½ T dijon mustard
14 oz. soft tofu
1 T Parmesan cheese
2 t Worcestershire sauce

Method
1) Combine all ingredients in a blender or food processor.
2) Toss with crisp romaine leaves and freshly grated parmesan cheese.

Citrus Vinaigrette

Ingredients
2 T cider vinegar
1 T lemon juice
1 T orange juice
2 T minced onion
½ t sea salt, or to taste
¼ t black pepper
½ cup extra virgin olive oil

Method
1) Put vinegar, citrus juices, onion, salt and pepper in a bowl and whisk to combine
2) Slowly whisk in the olive oil.

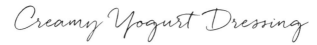

Creamy Yogurt Dressing

Ingredients

5 T white wine vinegar
4 T walnut oil
1/2 cup yogurt, sour cream or crème fraiche
1 t Dijon mustard
8 T extra-virgin olive oil
Handful of chopped parsley leaves
Sea salt and freshly ground black pepper to taste

Method

1) Combine all the ingredients in a bowl and whisk until combined.

2) Season to taste and adjust with a little more vinegar if needed.

Ginger Asian Vinaigrette

Ingredients

3 T rice vinegar
1 large piece fresh ginger
2/3 cup extra-virgin olive oil
1 T sesame oil;
Sea salt and freshly ground black pepper to taste

Method

1) Peel the piece of ginger and grate with a box grater. Then squeeze the grated ginger to obtain about 1 T ginger juice. Discard the grated ginger.

2) Whisk together in a bowl the ginger juice and the rice vinegar.

3) Whisk while incorporating the olive oil.

4) Add the sesame oil and season to taste.

Honey Lime Dressing

Ingredients

Juice of 1 lime
3 T olive oil
1 T honey
Sea salt and fresh cracked pepper, to taste
1 clove garlic, minced
Dash of cayenne pepper

Especially good over a summer salad of:

1 pint grape tomatoes
1 ripe avocado
2 ears of fresh sweet corn
2 T fresh cilantro, chopped

Italian Dressing

Ingredients

1½ cups tomato juice
⅓ cup plus 2 T red wine vinegar
2 minced garlic cloves (1 T)
2 t dried oregano or 2 T fresh oregano, minced
2 t dried basil or 2 T fresh basil, minced
¼ t black pepper (or to taste)
3 T olive oil
3 T grated Parmesan cheese

Method

Combine all ingredients and mix by hand.

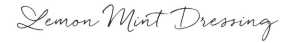

Lemon Mint Dressing

Ingredients

1 cup yogurt
2 T honey
1/8 cup of fresh mint
1/8 cup of fresh lemon juice
1/4 t salt
Dash of pepper
Lemon zest

Method

1) Combine all ingredients in a blender.

Lemon Vinaigrette

Ingredients

3 T fresh lime or lemon juice
1/2 t Dijon mustard, optional
3/4 cup extra-virgin olive oil
Sea salt and freshly ground black pepper to taste

Method

1) Combine all the ingredients except the oil.
2) Add the oil slowly while whisking vigorously. Using a blender will help to emulsify the vinaigrette.
3) Shake well before using.

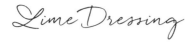

Lime Dressing

Ingredients

1/4 cup fresh lime juice (made from about 2 limes)
zest from 1 lime
1 T olive oil
1/4 t cinnamon
1/8 t paprika

Method

Blend and serve.

Orange & Rosemary Vinaigrette

Ingredients

3 T fresh lime or lemon juice
1/2 t Dijon mustard (optional)
3/4 cup extra-virgin olive oil
Grated zest and juice of 1 orange
1 t chopped rosemary
Sea salt and freshly ground black pepper to taste

Technique

Prepare like a traditional lemon vinaigrette and add the grated zest and juice of one orange and 1 t chopped rosemary. Let infuse overnight for a better taste.

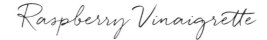

Ingredients
½ cup water
1T honey
½ T arrowroot or cornstarch
¼ cup raspberry vinegar
½ t stone ground mustard
½ cup fresh raspberries

Method
1) Combine water and raspberries. Blend.
2) Add the raspberry "water," honey and arrowroot in a small sauce pan and cook over low heat to thicken.
3) Whisk raspberry vinegar and mustard into dressing and mix well.
4) Cool or chill before using.

Raspberry Walnut Vinaigrette

Ingredients
3 T raspberry vinegar
1/2 t Dijon mustard (optional)
3/4 cup walnut oil
2 T chopped walnuts
Sea salt and freshly ground black pepper to taste

Method
1) Proceed like you would for a classic vinaigrette. Add the chopped walnuts at the end.

Sesame Ginger Dressing

Ingredients

1/2 cup rice wine vinegar
1/4 cup water
1/4 cup yellow miso paste
1/4 cup chopped green onions
2 T honey
2 T minced and peeled fresh ginger
2 T tamari sauce (or soy sauce)
4 T olive oil
2 T sesame oil

Method

1) Combine first three ingredients in a bowl, whisking until smooth.

2) Stir in onions and all remaining ingredients.

3) Store in airtight container in refrigerator.

Thai Peanut Dressing

Ingredients

2 T smooth peanut butter, preferably natural
2 t fresh lemon juice
2 t low sodium soy sauce
¼ cup plain yogurt
2 t honey
1 T rice vinegar
Pinch red pepper flakes (more, if you like)
1 t finely minced garlic (optional)

Method

1) Whisk all ingredients together except the yogurt.

2) Fold in the yogurt.

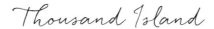

Thousand Island

Ingredients
¼ cup soft tofu
2 T plain soy milk
2 T ketchup
¼ t onion powder
¼ t granulated garlic
2 T dill pickle relish

Method
1) Purée everything except the dill pickle relish until smooth.
2) Add dill pickle relish and mix thoroughly.

Tomato Vinaigrette

Ingredients
Lemon Vinaigrette (see recipe)
4 oz cherry tomatoes
1 crushed clove of garlic

Method
Add all ingredients in a blender and process to a smooth purée. Thin it with a little water if necessary.

This is also good on grilled chicken or fish.

Warm Dressing

Ingredients

1 crushed garlic clove
1 finely chopped shallot or small onion
7 T olive oil or clarified butter
1/2 cup peeled, diced and finely diced tomatoes
Juice of 1/2 lemon
2 t chopped basil;

Method

1) Place the garlic and chopped shallot or onion in a pot with the oil or clarified butter and heat the ingredients until soft without frying.

2) Add the tomatoes and cook at a low heat for about 5 minutes and then add the lemon juice and chopped basil and stir.

3) Season to taste and serve the sauce hot.

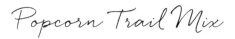

Popcorn Trail Mix

Ingredients

2 cups popped popcorn (preferably unsalted)
3/4 cup roasted almonds or roasted peanuts (preferably unsalted)
3/4 cup unsweetened dried banana chips
3/4 cup fruit-juice sweetened dried cranberries

Method

Combine all ingredients in a medium bowl. Divide between 8 small
storage containers. Trail mix will keep about 5 days.

Super Food Pudding

This Superfood Pudding is a delicious way to get lots of goodies into your diet, and best of all, its chocolate!

Ingredients
¼ cup of Chia Seeds
¼ cup of Goji Berries
1 T Cacao Powder
1 cup Unsweetened Vanilla Almond Milk

Method
Mix all the ingredients together in a bowl, and let it sit in the fridge for at least 30 minutes. The goji berries and chia seeds will absorb most of the liquid and become full of flavor, leaving you with a delicious, healthy, chocolate pudding!

Super Food Pudding

Why is this pudding so good for you?

Chia Seeds: Chia seeds have three times the amount of calcium than a glass of milk, more Omega 3 fatty acids than salmon, are low in saturated fat, and contain no cholesterol! Chia seeds also deliver 42% of your recommended daily value of fiber in a single serving, which is key for aiding digestion and promoting weight loss. Chia also absorbs up to twelve times its own weight and expands to curb your appetite, which reduces caloric intake.

Goji Berries: Goji berries have compounds rich in Vitamin A that may have anti-aging benefits, help boost immune function, protect vision, and even help prevent heart disease. Some studies suggest that goji berries may boost brain health by promoting calmness, happiness, better quality of sleep, and feelings of good health.

Cacao Powder: Chocolate is not just a guilty pleasure! Its bad reputation as a junk food should be more accurately attributed to the harmful effects of commercial processing and refining techniques, and the other ingredients commonly added, such as white sugar. Cacao in its unprocessed state is rich in nutrients, and has an enormous 10% antioxidant concentration level, which is ten times as high as blueberries!

Almond Milk: A serving of almonds provides an excellent source of vitamin E, and a good source of protein and fiber. (Higher than any other tree nut!) Plus, they're naturally low in saturated fat and cholesterol-free. Almond milk contains no lactose, making it easy to digest and the perfect alternative for those suffering from lactose intolerance. Try to buy unsweetened, because even though this milk is amazing for you, certain brands will add a lot of sugar. You can even make your own almond milk!

Milk and Honey Foot Bath

This foot bath is perfect to soothe tired and sore feet. The milk helps replenish dry skin and reduce irritation, and the cinnamon helps stimulate circulation.

Ingredients
3-5 T honey
1 t vanilla extract
2 t baking soda
1 t ground cinnamon
1/2 cup orange juice
1 cup whole milk

Directions
1) Mix ingredients.
2) Fill tub with warm water and stir in the mixture.
3) Let your feet soak for 10-15 minutes.

Exfoliating Sugar Scrub

Sugar scrubs are more gentle than other scrubs, and they exfoliate without damaging your skin – keeping it smooth and moisturized.

Ingredients
1 cup brown sugar
1/3 cup almond oil
1 t liquid vitamin E
1 t vanilla extract

Directions
1) Combine ingredients, adding in sugar last.
2) Use in the shower and apply in a circular motion.

Red Grape Face Mask

The grapes and cranberries have vitamins A and C, which help guard against sun damage. Additionally, this mask may help reverse some discoloration from aging.

Ingredients
1 cup seedless red grapes
1 cup fresh cranberries
2 t grapefruit juice
1 envelope unflavored gelatin

Directions
1) Mash up and mix ingredients together by hand or in a blender until it becomes a paste.
2) Chill for 45 minutes until it thickens.
3) Let it sit for 10 minutes and apply to clean skin.
4) Leave it on for 15 minutes and clean off with warm water.

Organic Sugar Scrub

Ingredients
1 cup organic cane or brown sugar
1/3 cup almond or organic olive oil.

Optional: If you would like your scrub scented, place drops of an essential oil. You can find organic pure essential oils at your local health foods store.
Note: If you would like to make a tougher scrub for exfoliation of areas like feet, simply substitute Epson Salt for sugar.

Directions
1) In a medium bowl, mix sugar with drops of essential oil, mixing a few drops at a time until it is scented to your liking.
2) Mix in your almond or olive oil.

Cinnamon and Ginger Sea Salt Scrub

Ingredients
    1 cup of sea salt
    ½ t of ground ginger
    ½ t ground cinnamon
    1 cup olive or almond oil

Directions
1) In a medium bowl, mix salt, ginger and cinnamon.
2) Mix in your almond or olive oil.

Oatmeal and Almond Milk Scrub

Ingredients
    ½ cup baking soda
    ½ cup oatmeal
    2 bags of green tea - cut open bag to empty contents into bowl
    1 cup almond milk

Optional: If you would like your scrub scented, place drops of an essential oil. You can find organic pure essential oils at your local health foods store.

Directions
1) In a medium bowl, mix dry ingredients with drops of essential oil, mixing a few drops at a time until it is scented to your liking.
2) Mix in your almond or olive oil.

Honey Banana Leg Mask

Ingredients

1 T almond or avocado oil
1 T Shea oil
1 banana
1 T honey
3 drops of peppermint oil
4 T unscented body lotion

Directions

1) Crush the banana with a fork until well mashed.

2) Place in a bowl, add remaining ingredients and stir until well blended.

Nourishing Lemon Hand & Foot Sugar Scrub

Ingredients

1½ T honey
3 T sugar
Juice of ½-1 lemon (depending on the size)

Directions

1) Mix all ingredients in a bowl.

2) Exfoliate hands and feet with the scrub, and let it sit on the skin for 5 minutes.

3) Wash and apply a replenishing cream.

Anti-Aging Yogurt & Honey Facial

Ingredients
1 cup yogurt
1 T oats
1 T honey
Rose water (available at any pharmacy)

Directions
1) Mix yogurt with the honey and oats in a bowl.
2) Apply the mixture on your face using massaging motions. Let stand 5 minutes.
3) Wash with cool water and apply rose water with a cotton pad.
4) Finish with your favorite face cream.

Firming Avocado/Cucumber Masque Recipe

Ingredients
1 organic avocado, mashed
3 t dry green clay
½ organic cucumber, pureed
1 t freshly squeezed lemon juice

Directions
1) Mix all ingredients in mixing bowl, allow to chill in refrigerator for up to an hour.
2) Apply a dense layer on face and allow to dry for 15-20 minutes.
3) Wipe skin clean with warm washcloth, splash will cool water and pat dry.

Brown Sugar Scrub

Ingredients

1 cup brown sugar
½ cup sweetened almond oil
1 t vitamin E
1 t vanilla extract

Directions

1) Simply combine all the liquid ingredients together, then mix in the sugar.
2) Use in the shower, rubbing it into your skin in circular motions.
3) Rinse sugar off (don't wash the oil off though!) and your skin should be silky smooth and well-moisturized.

Simple Rosemary Citrus Body Polish

Ingredients

2 T crushed rosemary
¼ cup natural sea salt
¼ cup oil (grape seed, coconut, etc.)
1 t fresh squeezed lemon juice
1 T honey

Mix together and enjoy!

Simple Face Steaming

To achieve maximum benefits of any mask, an initial gentle steaming of the face is recommended, which is as easy as boiling a pot of water!

Just toss a few bags of chamomile tea or lavender into a pot of boiling water and pour the water into a bowl or sink. Tent your head with a towel to capture the steam for several minutes, then proceed with a mask suitable for your skin type.

Mask for Oily Skin

- Mix 1 egg white with 1 tablespoon fresh lemon juice and 1 tablespoon plain yogurt.
- Apply to a cleansed face and let dry for 20 minutes.
- Remove with warm water and follow with a moisturizer.

Mask for Combination Skin

- Separate 1 egg and beat the white and the yolk separately.
- Cover the dry areas with the yolk and the oily parts with the white.
- Leave on for 20 minutes and remove with warm water, then follow with a moisturizer.

Mask for Dry Skin

- Mix 1 tablespoon wheat germ oil with ½ mashed avocado.
- Apply to skin and relax for 20-30 minutes as it nourishes the skin. The vitamin E in avocado will do wonders for the skin.
- Remove with a damp, soft washcloth or a warm splash of water.

Avocado Olive Oil Split-End Treatment

Olive oil is incredibly moisturizing for dry, damaged hair and will also make your hair more silky and shiny. Avocado is also known to contain many nutrients and vitamins conducive to healthy skin and hair.

Ingredients
1 avocado, pitted and skinned
2 T egg whites
3 T olive oil

Directions
1) Mash up the avocado and mix in the egg whites and olive oil. Whip until you obtain a creamy consistency like conditioner.
2) Apply to your hair, cover with a shower cap and let sit for 45 minutes to an hour.
3) Rinse thoroughly and wash hair with a mild, natural shampoo to get the mixture out but let the nutrients keep working.

Papaya Yogurt Hair Mask

Papaya is rich in protein and amino acids, which can help to make hair stronger. Mixed with plain yogurt, it makes a luxurious hair mask that will make your hair silky smooth and strong.

Ingredients
1 papaya, de-seeded and skinned
½ cup plain yogurt

Directions
1) Cut the papaya in half and scoop out the seeds, then use a knife to remove the skin.
2) Mash it up with a fork and then mix in the yogurt, whipping it until you obtain a smooth consistency.
3) Apply to hair like conditioner, and put on a shower cap and let it sit for 45 minutes to an hour.
4) Rinse thoroughly.

Epsom Salt Bath

Taking an Epsom salt bath can be both relaxing and rewarding.

Epsom salt is not truly a salt. It's a mineral composed of magnesium and sulfate. When soaking in a bath with Epsom salt, your body is able to absorb these beneficial ingredients.

Stress can lower your body's level of magnesium. By absorbing magnesium through an Epsom salt bath you can increase your magnesium levels again, which in turn can increase your production of serotonin (a chemical in the brain associated with feelings of relaxation). Magnesium can also help reduce irritability and improve sleep and concentration.

The sulfates found in Epsom salts can help draw out the toxins in your body. By bathing in an Epsom salt bath your skin is able to absorb the beneficial sulfates while eliminating some toxins from your body, and even decrease puffiness.

Directions
1) Fill your tub with warm water.
2) Relax for about 10-20 minutes or so.
3) When done, get up slowly and rinse in cool water.
4) After your bath, use as natural and gentle a product as you can. After your Epsom salt bath your pores tend to be open, which makes it easy for your body to absorb any chemicals or harsh ingredients that may be in your body products. Also, make sure to stay hydrated by drinking water before and after your bath.

Try adding a few drops of your favorite essential oil. Lavender is very popular for its relaxing effects. Try spearmint and rosemary for some added energy. Or try orange oil for an uplifting citrus bath.

Epsom Salt Foot Bath

To ease achy feet, soften skin, and reduce calluses, add ½ a cup of Epsom salt in a small tub of warm water.

Soak your feet for about 20 minutes or so.

10 Homemade Facial Tips

1) A good facial needn't be expensive -- an egg white whipped up nice and frothy will work wonders. Leave it on for 10 minutes, rinse with cool water and pat dry.

2) For a great facial toner, mix a few drops of lemon juice with yogurt, but make sure you keep it away from your eyes.

3) Try an oatmeal facial combining one egg yolk with 1 tbsp of cooked oatmeal, I tbsp of honey and 1/8 tsp of lemon juice. Pat gently on face, keeping away for your eyes and rinse off after 20 minutes.

4) Moisturize your skin by blending half a mashed banana and half an avocado with 1 tsp of honey and leave on your face for 20 minutes.

5) Tone up and moisturize tired skin with a carrot juice facial. Blend 2 tsp of carrot juice, an egg white (for oily skin) or an egg yolk (for dry skin) and 1 tbsp of honey. Leave it on for 20 minutes before rinsing.

6) Need an astringent? Grapefruit juice is excellent or if you would rather not use something quite so acidic, try using buttermilk over your face, allow to dry and rinse off with cool water

7) Blemishes will fade away with frequent dabs of lemon juice applied to them.

8) Dead skin will peel off elbows knees, feet and your face when massaged liberally with mayonnaise.

9) Pack your bags (eye bags, that is) with dampened gauze squares filled with raw grated potato. This will temporarily eliminate puffiness around the eyes. Refresh tired eyes with slices of cucumber; keep them in place about 10 minutes.

Lime Sugar Scrub

The acid in the fruit's juice sloughs off dry patches.

Ingredients
Juice of 2 limes
.5 cup brown sugar
4 T coconut oil

Directions
1) In a small bowl, whisk the lime juice and sugar until it is free of clumps.
2) Add the coconut oil one tablespoon at a time to thicken.
3) In the shower, apply all over your body in small circles. Rinse.

Coconut Oil Hair Conditioner

If you're looking for a deep hair conditioner that's chemical-free, look no further than virgin coconut oil. It's one of the best hair conditioners and if it's virgin and organic, it's chemical free and natural.

Coconut oil is one of the best natural treatments for hair. It's been used by indigenous people around the world, from South America, Africa, India and Asia.

It brings back the softness to your hair thanks to its bountiful medium chain triglycerides (or fatty acids).

While other conditioners work from the outside in, coconut oil is able to work from the inside out. It's an excellent conditioner and helps in the re-growth of damaged hair as it stimulates blood circulation in the scalp. Here's why.

Coconut oil keeps your hair full (and won't make it fall out).

It's well established that coconut oil is high in antioxidants, which helps to prevent free radical damage to the body, including heat and environmental damage.

Most conditioners on the market use processed vegetable oils that actually create free radicals and are completely stripped of their original antioxidant power, causing hair to lose protein and fall out over time. One of the reasons behind hair loss is microbial action on the scalp and hair roots.

So, to protect hair against them, what we need is an antimicrobial agent. Lauric acid in Coconut Oil is one of them. It's basically a triglyceride which yields a monoglyceride called Monolaurin, an excellent antimicrobial.

Coconut oil provides relief from dandruff.

Coconut oil nourishes the scalp because the oil is a natural antifungal, antimicrobial, antibacterial and has soothing properties. It can also offer relief from dandruff conditions. Dandruff is often caused by an internal fungal condition that reaches the scalp, called candida overgrowth. With regular use, coconut oil can kill the fungus in the scalp and dandruff issues can be eliminated. Then, you can say get rid of chemically oriented dandruff shampoos that add to your body's toxic burden of chemicals.

Coconut oil is readily absorbed into the skin and when applied to the scalp, it is absorbed into the blood for a quick dose of a powerful natural antifungal, antiviral and antibacterial which builds immunity. For additional benefits, the oil can be applied to the entire body instead of using chemical-based lotions.

Just apply a teaspoon or two from head to toe after your shower, rub it in, and let it absorb a few minutesbefore toweling off.

Coconut oil provides deep conditioning.

Coconut oil's fatty acids have a unique molecular structure that penetrates easily into the hair shaft. A hair is just like a hose or a tube. It is hollow from inside. Coconut oil fully penetrates this hollow space (the hair shaft).

This allows the nourishing oil to penetrate your hair's shaft - and literally brings deep conditioning from within reducing the loss of internal moisture.

For deep hair conditioning, use a teaspoon or two on damp hair and leave it in as long as possible. Coconut oil is solid at room temperature so warm it to liquefy it. Make sure to massage the scalp to allow blood circulation. Once you have saturated all of your hair, wrap a towel or something around your head and leave it for one to two hours to see results right away.

Then fully rinse you hair and wash with shampoo. Note that coconut oil can stain fabric, so be sure to protect your clothes and bedding if sleeping with it on your head overnight. This deep conditioning can be done as often as once a week and you may need to wash your hair a couple times to remove all of it.

Work Cited

Sugar and Addiction

1. Abundance of Fructose Not Good for the Liver, Heart. Harvard Medical School, Sept. 2011. Web. <http://www.health.harvard.edu/newsletters/Harvard_Heart_Letter/2011/September/abundance-of-fructose-not-good-for-the-liver-heart>.

2. Lenoir, M., F. Serre, and SH Ahmed. "Intense Sweetness Surpasses Cocaine Reward." Plos (2007): n. pag. Web.

3. Parker, Hilary. "A Sweet Problem: Princeton Researchers Find That High-fructose Corn Syrup Prompts Considerably More Weight Gain." Princeton University. Trustees of Princeton University, 22 Mar. 2010. Web. 17 Oct. 2014.

4. "Methamphetamine Abuse and Addiction." NIDA Research Report. NIH Publication No. 06-4210 (2006).

5. "Kenneth Blum." Wikipedia. Wikimedia Foundation, n.d. Web. <http://en.wikipedia.org/wiki/Kenneth_Blum>.

6. "Scripps Research Study Shows Compulsive Eating Shares Same Addictive Biochemical Mechanism with Cocaine, Heroin Abuse." The Scripps Research Institute, 23 Mar. 2010. Web. <http://www.scripps.edu/news/press/2010/20100329.html>.

7. Koob, G. F. "Alcoholism: Allostasis and Beyond." Alchoholism, Clinical and Experimental Research (2003): 232-43. National Center for Biotechnology Information. U.S. National Library of Medicine, Feb. 2003. Web. <http://www.ncbi.nlm.nih.gov/pubmed/12605072>.

8. Fleming, A. "Food Addiction: Does It Really Exist?" Web log post. The Guardian, 20 Aug. 2013. Web. <http://www.theguardian.com/lifeandstyle/wordofmouth/2013/aug/20/food-addiction-exist-fat-sugar>.

9. Ren, X., and J. G. Ferreira. "Nutrient Selection in the Absence of Taste Recep-

tor Signaling." Journal of Neuroscience (2010): 8012-023. Print.

10. DesMaisons, Kathleen. The Sugar Addict's Total Recovery Program. New York: Ballantine Pub. Group, 2000. Print.

Step 1: Join the Breakfast Club

11. Leidy, H. J., R. J. Lepping, C. R. Savage, and C. T. Harris. "Neural Responses to Visual Food Stimuli after a Normal vs. Higher Protein Breakfast in Breakfast-skipping Teens: A Pilot FMRI Study." Obesity (2011).

12. Miller, Kelli. "Skip Breakfast, Get Fat." WebMD, 15 June 2009. Web. <http://www.webmd.com/diet/news/20090615/skip-breakfast-get-fat?_sm_au_=iSH0qmR5Q5WHRj76>.

13. "National Weight Control Registry Facts." Research Findings. National Weight Control Registry, 18 Oct. 2014. Web. <http://www.nwcr.ws/Research/>.

14. "Eating Eggs for Breakfast Helps Reduce Calorie Consumption throughout the Day by 18 Percent." Eating Eggs for Breakfast Helps Reduce Calorie Consumption throughout the Day by 18 Percent. Phys.org, 06 Apr. 2010. Web. 18 Oct. 2014. <http://phys.org/news189782584.html>.

15. Vander Wal, J. S., A. Gupta, P. Khosla, and N. V. Dhurandhar. "Egg Breakfast Enhances Weight Loss." Nature.com. Nature Publishing Group, 05 Aug. 2008. Web. 18 Oct. 2014. <http://www.nature.com/ijo/journal/v32/n10/full/ijo2008130a.html>.

Step 4: Get Up and Go

16. Garland, Theodore, Jr. "The Biological Control of Voluntary Exercise, Spontaneous Physical Activity and Daily Energy Expenditure in Relation to Obesity: Human and Rodent Perspectives." The Journal of Experimental Biology, 04 Nov. 2010. Web. 18 Oct. 2014. <http%3A%2F%2Fjeb.biologists.org%2Fcontent%2F214%2F2%2F206.long%3F_sm_>.

17. Wang, G. J. "Brain Dopamine and Obesity." National Center for Biotechnology Information. U.S. National Library of Medicine, 03 Feb. 2001. Web. 18 Oct.

2014. <http://www.ncbi.nlm.nih.gov/pubmed/11210998>.

18. Spilner, Maggie. "A Step Ahead Of Stress." Prevention. N.p., Nov. 2011. Web. 18 Oct. 2014. <http://www.prevention.com/fitness/fitness-tips/reduce-stress-walking-exercise>.

Step 5: Slash the Sugar

19. "Principles of Harm Reduction." Harm Reduction Coalition. Web. 17 Oct. 2014. <http://harmreduction.org/about-us/principles-of-harm-reduction/>.

20. Amen, Daniel G. Change Your Brain, Change Your Life: The Breakthrough Program for Conquering Anxiety, Depression, Obsessiveness, Anger, and Impulsiveness. New York: Times, 2000. Print.

21. Taheri, Shahrad, Ling Lin, Diane Austin, Terry Young, and Emmanuel Mignot. "Short Sleep Duration Is Associated with Reduced Leptin, Elevated Ghrelin, and Increased Body Mass Index." National Center for Biotechnology Information. U.S. National Library of Medicine, 07 Dec. 2004. Web. 18 Oct. 2014. <http://www.ncbi.nlm.nih.gov/pmc/articles/PMC535701/>.

22. Speigel, K. "Sleep Curtailment in Healthy Young Men Is Associated with Decreased Leptin Levels, Elevated Ghrelin Levels, and Increased Hunger and Appetite." National Center for Biotechnology Information. U.S. National Library of Medicine, 07 Dec. 2004. Web. 18 Oct. 2014. <http://www.ncbi.nlm.nih.gov/pubmed/15583226>.

23. Nedeltcheva, A. V. "Sleep Curtailment Is Accompanied by Increased Intake of Calories from Snacks." The American Journal of Clinical Nutrition, Jan. 2009. Web. 18 Oct. 2014. <http://ajcn.nutrition.org/content/89/1/126.full>.

Step 6: Love Yourself Silly

24. Scheve, Tom. "What Are Endorphins?" HowStuffWorks. HowStuffWorks. com, n.d. Web. 18 Oct. 2014. <http://science.howstuffworks.com/life/endorphins1.htm>.

46801361R00181

Made in the USA
San Bernardino, CA
16 March 2017